SUBLIMINALLY EXPOSED

Be advised, cautioned and forewarned:

This book may forever change the way you see and feel about your significant other, best friend and boss. All of your relationships and the decisions you make will be affected to some degree by the words you are about to read.

SUBLIMINALLY
EXPOSED

Shocking truths about your hidden desires
in mating, dating and communicating.
Use Cautiously.

Steven H. Dayan, MD

NEW YORK

SUBLIMINALLY EXPOSED

Shocking truths about your hidden desires in mating, dating and communicating.
Use Cautiously.

ISBN 978-1-61448-586-5 paperback
ISBN 978-1-61448-587-2 eBook
Library of Congress Control Number: 2013934149

Morgan James Publishing
The Entrepreneurial Publisher
5 Penn Plaza, 23rd Floor,
New York City, New York 10001
(212) 655-5470 office • (516) 908-4496 fax
www.MorganJamesPublishing.com

Interior Design by:
Bonnie Bushman
bonnie@caboodlegraphics.com

In an effort to support local communities, raise awareness and funds, Morgan James Publishing donates a percentage of all book sales for the life of each book to Habitat for Humanity Peninsula and Greater Williamsburg.

Get involved today, visit
www.MorganJamesBuilds.com.

Habitat
for Humanity®
Peninsula and
Greater Williamsburg
Building Partner

True advancement in human nature arises from the fringes of where different fields of thought merge.
Steven H. Dayan

TABLE OF CONTENTS

PREFACE

"Dr. Dayan, we're here because we want to see for ourselves if it's true—the results you show don't seem possible; the word on the street is that you're altering patient' photographs, testimonies and faking your outcomes."

This is how three medical school students from University of Illinois greeted me when they came to my office to explore for themselves the approach that was making such a groundbreaking impact on both modern and traditional cosmetic techniques. They had heard claims about my method and skill set that allow a person to instantly look and feel more attractive and had seen the before-and-after photos demonstrating a significant improvement yet what exactly was done remains elusive to the untrained observer. Evidently the pictures looked too good to be true, just like the patient testimonials they'd been reading.

Contrary to conventional wisdom, the desire to be attractive transcends social, economic and cultural boundaries. In this book I will describe the life-changing experiences of people of all ages, from teenagers with cleft lips who feel "branded" in society and after treatment begin to live fully for the first time to elderly women who want to recapture feelings of youthfulness. I'll tell the stories of victims of domestic violence who made surprising discoveries about how to heal the emotional scars that lie deeper than the physical ones, of prisoners who wanted to gain control of their lives with a boost of self-confidence as well as a traveler from a West African nation who sought a way to achieve higher social status. All of them raised their self-esteem through an improvement in their appearance. I am fascinated by the impact appearance has

Once you grasp the basics on this journey into the primitive world of human programming which you are about to embark, there will be no turning back—your perception of yourself and others will never be the same.

on our self-worth, how it affects the judgment and treatment we receive and the critical role it plays in driving human kind forward.

I wrote this book to reveal that what I teach, think and do is based on real, palpable aspects of human behavior and biology. What I tell you will likely make you rethink the way you put on make-up, how you walk into a room and why you and those with whom you interact make decisions and behave the way you do. But be advised, cautioned and forewarned: this book may forever change the way you see and feel about your boss, best friend and/or significant other. For some this will mean a deeper, more complete and inspired relationship, and for others the opportunity to seal the end of a lifeless union.

All of your relationships and the decisions you make will be affected to some degree by the words you are about to read.

Once you grasp the basics on this journey into the primitive world of human programming which you are about to embark, there will be no turning back—your perception of yourself and others will never be the same.

I have always been intrigued by the friction that occurs at the intersection of various fields of study. Most academics are focused in one area, but many of the greatest breakthroughs in human advancement and thinking happen at the crossroads of multiple disciplines of science and the humanities. From Plato and Einstein to the more recently departed Steve Jobs, the desire to push thinking to another level based on the merging of specific areas of science with the aesthetic paths of art has always captivated me. The origins of my theories that I reveal in this book are based on the unique culmination of experiences from three areas of study: Evolutionary biology, Neuropsychiatry and Aesthetic medicine.

> Sorely missing from plastic surgery training is an introspective exploration of what makes someone feel ideal and why.

During college I majored in biology and was introduced to anthropology and the evolutionary sciences, two fields that continue to stimulate me. As a burgeoning sculptor I was trained to visualize the three-dimensional ideals of facial beauty and create forms that meet the designs of the divine proportions. And as a medical student possessing a long fascination with the workings of the human mind, I found myself contemplating a career in psychiatry. My Type "A" personality, however, seemed better suited for a surgical field. And aesthetic medicine, plastic surgery in particular with a specialization in the face seemed to be the perfect fit for satisfying my intellectual pursuits and providing an outlet for my creative aspiration.

Having now been in practice for more than twelve years, I have had the privilege of witnessing the relationships, innermost fears, and desires of over 40,000 people. I have interviewed each of them in depth and been fortunate to treat them with surgery, non-surgical aesthetic treatments or, in many cases, nothing other than conversation. Each patient has given me the opportunity to observe and learn what can be accomplished within ourselves and in our relationships when we make a shift in our self-esteem. And I can now unequivocally state that more than any other field of study, facial plastic surgery allows a scientist the closest and most practical position from which to experience the intersection of beauty, evolutionary biology and the human mind. However, until now there has been little to no writing or research on this incredibly important union of forces.

Perhaps the problem is that observing art is more of a personal experience, the biological and psychological sciences miss on capturing every day clinical experiences, and training in plastic surgery has traditionally been too one dimensional. Like terracotta sculpting, plastic surgery has always been based on inanimate designs of the ideal, but sorely missing from the training is an introspective exploration of what makes someone feel ideal and why. As a surgeon with artistic skill I knew I could design and even make a face beautiful, but I wanted to know more. I was determined to grasp the essence of beauty and attraction by exploring how science, art and clinical practice could come together to answer the mystifying questions about human desire:

1. Why are ideally proportioned faces perceived as beautiful?
2. How does being beautiful affect both the conscious and subconscious mind of the individual?
3. Why are beautiful people often perceived as better and gain advantages in life?
4. Why is there such a stark difference between being beautiful and being attractive?
5. Why does being beautiful have so little to do with being happy?
6. What is the correlation between being beautiful and making a positive first impression?
7. How do sex and our sexual features intertwine with beauty and attractiveness?
8. Why do we feel euphoric when our brains are stimulated by beauty?
9. How does our irresistible, insatiable drive for beauty affect every decision we make in life?
10. And finally, when did plastic surgery go wrong?

Plastic surgery has been taught at a shallow, flat and simple level rather than in a manner that embraces its deeper, more visceral and consequential effects. This field is not a matter of paint by numbers or cut and paste; plastic surgery affects people's lives in ways that may not be well illustrated or understood because the professionals may not always ask the right questions. Not long after I opened my practice I recognized a void—something else at the core of plastic surgery was dictating outcomes, an unexplained, poorly understood but critical component to being attractive: the human element. I became convinced that my profession needed to make a careful evaluation of what makes someone appear and feel attractive and integrate that knowledge into clinical practice.

Being intellectually curious I started to read deeper and explore further the sciences of human evolution and neuropsychiatry to better understand how the mind interprets beauty and why we gain so much pleasure from it. I also studied the artistic masters and, yearning for further inspiration, traveled to places of beauty to understand it from the perspective of different cultures. I wanted to find the link or common denominator that defined what all human beings find attractive regardless of outside influences or methods for achieving it. I travelled to Italy, France, Iceland, China, Thailand, Vietnam, Cambodia, Bali, India, Brazil, Morocco, Galapagos Islands, the Middle East and more. I explored pyramids, statues, caves and remote islands where I observed, read, questioned and wrote. And as I viewed art, customs and traditions from these vastly different worlds and immersed myself in the study of others, I started to see similarities where others often declare differences. A hazy picture became increasingly clear. I began to grasp the thread that weaves through all of us, regardless of color, creed, education or society. I started formulating thoughts into something tangible that could be crafted and delivered into practice. And soon I came up with new ways of thinking that resulted in more focused and purposeful techniques for cosmetic treatments that went beyond treating the physical to affecting the very depths of the human soul, tapping into the essence and spirit of humanity.

> I came up with new ways of thinking that resulted in more focused and purposeful techniques for cosmetic treatments that went beyond treating the physical to affecting the very depths of the human soul.

The further I advanced the better I became at applying these truths to my practice. It was as if a veil had been lifted and I was able to see something that was not there before. I could perceive a face as a window to the mind and instantly know what it takes to make someone not only appear more beautiful but feel more attractive. And as my thoughts crystallized and techniques purified I realized these advancements were counter to the orthodox wisdom of bigger, better and more dramatic plastic surgery. Instead, I was preaching about doing less. Beyond the mathematical formulas for defining beauty, my theories were based on the how and why subtle, strategic and covert cosmetic alterations to a face in turn alter our deeply subconscious perceptions.

I knew that colleagues would be uncomfortable with my ideas. How could they not? I was professing to make changes that can't be seen, or at least not to those who don't know what to look for. I suggested a retraining of

> Doubters arose, as they always do, but it's the skeptics who drive the creative types to prove their visions.

plastic surgeons to see the face differently and understand the interaction between the mind and the face. Doubters arose, as they always do, but it's the skeptics who drive the creative types to prove their visions. And as a scientist I knew I could not be true to myself or others until I validated my theories in exacting clinical trials, so I designed studies and tested my theories in trials that have subsequently been published in peer-reviewed journals.

The more I studied, probed and pushed the envelope, the more I uncovered. By melding the fields of neuropsychiatry, art, human evolution and cosmetic medicine, wonderful new ways to help people began to emerge. And not just for those of financial means, but all people—children with facial deformities, cancer sufferers, victims of domestic violence and the elderly all could potentially benefit from our findings. In essence we are on the cusp of a new field of study and medicine, a discipline that explores the relationship between self-esteem, health and aesthetics of the body.

I welcomed the three the young skeptics to my office that day because I was thrilled to learn that my ideas and practices were pushing people to question their assumptions about beauty and the field of plastic surgery. Their demand to know if our photographs were fake was the best proof to date that my revolutionary approach to attractiveness was working.

Our survival-motivated urges to eat and drink are well understood, but our equally primal instinct to be attracted to beauty and act on that desire has not been seriously addressed. For too long, the political, social, religious and moral overtones of a modern society have swept the subject under the rug. This book changes all that.

As you read ahead, I ask that you to take a very candid, honest and sometimes uncomfortable look at your primitive urges and drop any sense of moral superiority that makes you think you don't possess such drives. In that spirit of openness, explore how your desire for the pleasures of beauty influences your everyday decisions.

> This book is not about plastic surgery, Botox or the latest chemical peel; rather, it is focused on the human mind as it pertains to beauty, culture and evolution and the subtle yet incredibly forceful impact it has on your life.

This book is not about plastic surgery, Botox or the latest chemical peel; rather, it is focused on the human mind as it pertains to beauty, culture and evolution and the subtle yet incredibly forceful impact it has on your life. By the end, you may choose to change how you highlight your sexual "calling" features (attributes that accentuate your gender), completely alter your appearance or stop using cosmetics altogether. But regardless of your response, much like learning a new language, the knowledge and skills you are about to learn will open up a new world of possibilities for you. The social tools you gain can be used to better understand your motives and the decisions you make as well as influence the thoughts and actions of people close to you. Some may be tempted to use these tools with a deceitful intent and others may choose to not use them at all, but it is my hope that for most, a new understanding of who you are, where you come from and why you desire beauty will impart a positive and meaningful influence into your life.

INTRODUCTION

Picture this: After a long day at work, you and your friends decide to meet up for a drink. You are a just about to finish your cocktail when you see him walk into the room. He's tall and handsome with a chiseled jaw, deep-set eyes and a full head of hair. He confidently settles in at the bar, purposely unfastens the top button of his form-fitting designer suit and takes a sip of his martini. That's when he notices you and shoots you a playful smile. Your heart flutters as you play coy, avert your eyes and resume conversation with your friends. Knowing that he is watching, you get up and seductively make your way across the bar for another drink. As you sashay across the floor, you feel his eyes scanning your hips and moving up to your lips and eyes. As you sit down and fluidly cross your legs, you casually flip your head, allowing your hair to be tossed through the air. You gently turn your chin downward and direct your gaze towards his eyes. He gets the message and rises from his seat to move toward you.

While you were imagining that scene, real encounters very similar to it were happening all over the world, from a trendy club in Chicago to a dive bar in Berlin. Eyes met, hearts raced and potential mates were found. Using beauty to communicate a message matters! We may not like to admit it, but we all know and depend on it. The language of beauty is innate, consistent across all species and perhaps the rawest of all energies fueling evolution. It is evident in the above scenario that describes finding a partner, but an equally important parade of similar events occurs when interviewing for a job or encountering the in-laws for the first time. Regardless of the situation, the impression we make is lasting and consequential. Nature is big on efficiency, especially when it comes to sizing each other up.

It seems obvious that impressions would be based on physical traits, but it actually goes deeper than that, much deeper.

The ability to instantly sense danger, likability or aggressiveness in others has been hard-wired within the most primitive depths of our brains over tens of thousands years. This wiring follows our most basic neural pathways; I have discovered surprisingly simple actions that significantly alter the impression people project to others and in return how that impression changes the responses they receive. Project one type of signal, get one type of response. Project a different, more "attractive" signal, get a more positive reaction.

It's that basic. It's that quick. And it's that effective.

Nature created a set of basic human characteristics that shapes the first impression we convey, and you will become very familiar with them in the first half of this book. Once you understand the natural laws beneath our instinct to scan those qualities, you'll never look at people in the same way. You'll be able to predict people's actions and flow from one "aha!" moment to the next.

With that in mind, let's revisit the above chance encounter, but this time through the eyes of an evolutionary psychologist. First, as the well-dressed stranger studies the woman's walk, posture and how she carries herself, he is picking up certain clues about her breasts, buttocks and hips regarding her fertility. He notices her full lips, a powerful signal to suggest ovulation. Unblemished skin tips him off to her youngish age and underlying health. As she sits down and gently tosses her hair over her shoulder, she releases pleasant and genetically unique odors into the environment—a calling signal that seeps into his primitive brain. At that same subconscious level, he reads her lowered chin as a sign of her diminutive position, which indicates her need for assistance (vulnerability—another mark of youth). Altogether, those signals sum up that she's an ideal prospective mate.

> Where you end up in life may depend entirely on one chance encounter and the impression you make. The good news is you can use your knowledge of positive signals to set the laws of attraction in motion.

Meanwhile, the woman is processing the man's signals that exude confidence and masculinity. His chiseled jaw suggests high levels of testosterone (her primal brain knows this) and his tall, handsome demeanor imply that he has good genes. His suit jacket accentuates his physical prowess by emphasizing his overall level of fitness and forces her to notice that his upper torso is larger than his waist, indicating that he is strong and likely to be a good protector. All of those qualities stream together to form an impression that he is resourceful, both physically and emotionally. Then his eyes meet hers, piercing, direct and forceful. She may not realize it, but her brows are elevating and expanding and her pupils are maximally dilated, sure signs that she is interested.

As the man confidently walks up to her, his breathing rate increases in order to better inhale her pheromones. Her nose is also in the air testing for his smell to see if he is a genetic match. Everything about the rendezvous is serving a greater purpose—to signal the loud and clear message, "I have great genes!" This is the complicated yet lightning-fast process illustrating the power of beauty as the most primitive form of communication, an unconscious program running full-speed.

Where you end up in life may depend entirely on one chance encounter and the impression you make. The question I ask is why?

My passion is to teach, and regardless of the level, from grade through graduate school my mission is the same: I challenge the students to think, not regurgitate. I believe it is through education that barriers are broken down, prejudices are defeated and self-esteem is elevated. It is however my experiences at DePaul University where I seem to have the most impact. In my course on the *Science of Beauty*, on the first day of class I ask the students to define beauty. It's a difficult question to answer if you really think about it, and I always get very colorful responses. One of my students, whom I'll call James, was refreshingly direct about what he considered beautiful. James was an older student with a somewhat checkered past and he didn't care whom he offended when he blurted out, "Doc, it's all about the butt. I like my woman to have some junk in her trunk. Something extra to hold onto, you know?"

I told him I appreciated his candor, and I truly did admire his honesty (as evident by some of the eye rolls in class, however, not everyone felt the same about James' comments). We'll get to whether James was wrong or just a little indelicate about the truth in a later chapter, and you may be surprised by the answer.

I would bet that if we polled people on the street about their definition of beauty a few might click off some favorite traits like nice eyes, broad shoulders or long hair, but most would hide behind the politically correct answer that beauty is found on the inside. They may believe that, which is wonderful, but they also know that deep down they can't help but be attracted to certain characteristics and repelled by others.

Harnessing the Power of the First Impression

Many of the human instincts that developed to help our species survive aren't compatible with modern standards of behavior. We're taught to hold ourselves in check. This leads to the inner conflicts that Freud wrote about, but we can use the power of our instincts to our advantage, too. Once we know how to send out irresistibly positive/attractive signals, whether we're seeking a partner or trying to convince someone that we're the best person for the job, we can gain better understanding and more control of our lives.

When we make a step toward improving our attractiveness signal by getting a hairstyle and makeup that are perfectly appropriate for our facial structure, for example, we can expect more positive responses from others based not only on our physical appearance, but also on the energy surge we gain from our ramped-up self-esteem. Those enhancements are simple yet powerful adjustments that send positive signals that stimulate a positive response in the other person. A potential date may want to connect or a new employer may recruit us further into the fold.

Yet, if we go overboard with impression "enhancements" we can ignite the opposite response by tipping off someone's subconscious mind that we're trying to hide something, like bad genes, poor health or even deceit. It is the reason that women who wear excessive make-up are negatively perceived and that the comb over to a balding man is found highly unattractive. It is more beneficial to employ minor enhancement to what you already have than to try to be what you are not. Taking charge of the impression you project is easier than you think, thanks in part to the connection between the mind and our physiology. The mind has the ability to change the chemistry and other physical functioning of the body, and in medicine and science we call this the placebo effect. This effect can be as strong as many of our modern-day medical interventions, and we can learn to harness, hone and maximize our ability to use the mind to alter our first impression. When it comes to cosmetic alterations, whether a new fashion sense, hairstyle or a wrinkle removal treatment, I will show you how the placebo effect is likely to be as important as the products, procedure or treatment a person receives.

> Once we know how to send out irresistibly positive/attractive signals, whether we're seeking a partner or trying to convince someone that we're the best person for the job, we can gain more control of our lives.

The key is using the mind and the intervention synergistically. If a middle-aged adult wants to look more youthful and seeks out my assistance to remove forehead wrinkles, I can't realistically make the wrinkles go away by just telling her to visualize them gone and hoping the placebo effect works. That would be too simplistic. But after providing Botox, filler or laser treatments, I can reduce the wrinkles and prevent her brow from fully emoting anger. Studies show that once a person views her face with fewer wrinkles and is less efficient at emoting anger, she likely will feel better, thereby setting off a cascade of physiological and biochemical events that result in projecting a more youthful impression.

Likewise, there are minimal interventions—hairstyles, posture, clothing styles, makeup—we can all make that will increase the amount of likeability, friendliness or power we project. This, too, can be achieved without much effort, but it does require some insight. Once this particular insight into our instinctual responses is revealed and understood it becomes so blatantly obvious you will recognize signs and evidence of people engaging in it everywhere you look.

> There are minimal interventions we can all make that will increase the amount of likeability, friendliness or power we project.

By the end of this book you will have a solid grasp of how the brain processes impressions, which will open new doors of understanding. You will know why an eight-year-old boy gets teased by his classmates, for example, or how a local candidate got elected in spite of showing no leadership skills. You will see how our innate human preferences for certain physical characteristics show up consistently in cultures all over the world, such as the way buttocks signal a female's fertility. Larger buttocks may send that message in one culture and slimmer in another, but both are acting as the male signal catcher. Likewise, women everywhere are wired to value a resourceful male—in one culture they see this "resourcefulness" in a strong, lean upper body, while in another it's signaled by a fat wallet.

> To work with the foundations of our most basic drives instead of being unaware of or denying them is to give yourself a tremendous advantage in achieving what you want in life.

Over the eons of human existence, many social and political systems have been tried and tested, from democratic republics to tyrannical regimes. The morals and ethics of mating, marriage and child rearing have also varied widely based on the social, cultural and political factors of the times. However, evolution doesn't take these external forces into play. Nature's only concern is the survival of the fittest—from nurturing healthy bodies to nudging us toward mates that have the best odds of carrying on our genes.

That may sound too simplistic, but it's true. And to work *with* the foundations of our most basic drives instead of being unaware of or denying them is to give yourself a tremendous advantage in achieving what you want in life.

Whether you believe this system was instituted by intelligent design or by nature alone, the prevailing theory of evolution is one of natural selection. And it is within this raw system that human development can most easily be explained, including the workings of beauty, attraction and the first impression. I invite you to put any preconceived political, religious or cultural notions aside as you explore the science behind our behavior. If you are adamant that you don't care about how you look or that our concept of beauty is constructed by the media instead of our biology, I invite you to keep an open mind, too.

The truth is we're all concerned with the impression we make to some degree, even if that's limited to brushing our hair or making sure our socks match. This book will challenge you to look at yourself and others in a very broad and natural context, in which we are all, at the deepest level, spurred on by the same drives. To understand those drives is the first step in working them to your advantage.

It is important, however, to recognize I am not an anthropologist nor a psychologist but rather a medical doctor with an insatiable appetite for knowledge and on a mission to better understand the abstract relationship between beauty, self-esteem and human psyche. As a scientist I always ask, why. And it is this quest that has driven me deeper into these fields of study that are intimately related. My experience is real and practical; each day I work with cancer and trauma victims, elderly and the depressed all seeking aesthetic treatments as a means to regain psychological balance and normalcy. Additionally I see people of all ages desiring appearance enhancements in order to attract a new mate, job or impart a positive influence in their life. It is perhaps my ability to identify and unify the three fields of, evolutionary biology, neuropsychiatry and aesthetic medicine that has resulted in the success of my practice and the validation of my research. If you desire a more in-depth knowledge of the environmental and behavioral sciences please consider the references that have been listed at the back of the book. But, in this exploration of how evolution has shaped and impacted our relationship with beauty, I report only on research that has been conducted with proper scientific techniques. While at times the reports may seem to be skewed toward one gender, the fact is that of the more than 200 studies referenced in this book, sixty-six percent of them involve both men and women. It is also important to note that these studies deal with averages and norms. Research depends on overall trends and averages to define its results, but life is not that cut and dry. Keep that in mind when you feel that you or someone you know is the exception rather than the rule.

CHAPTER 1

THE WOMAN
IN WHITE

Why do we share the same attractiveness wiring as the Ancient Egyptians? How can the same blueprint for what's attractive apply to reindeer- and the average Joe or Jane on the street in Des Moines? What's nature been up to?

It's all about survival.

First impressions matter more than we care to admit, and making a positive impression often results in being singled out for favorable treatment. But it's not always easy to pinpoint that certain something in a person's appearance that projects a positive first impression. We often describe this mysterious trait as the X-Factor, especially when referencing actors, politicians, and business leaders who rise above the rest in stardom and success. But I call this quality the "F" Factor, because it captures the deep-seated messages about fertility and fear that underlie our immediate response to a first impression. Regardless of geography or point in history, all humans across all cultures have developed similar abilities to create and interpret positive and negative impressions.

We like to believe that we have evolved beyond our cave-dwelling ancestors, but when it comes to our most instinctive powers of perception—we haven't. The "F" Factor, which I divide into two modes, F1: The Fertility Factor and F2: The Fear Factor, is part of our most primal encoding. Learning how to read the "F" Factor and express it in ways that project the most positive first impression possible will change your life.

F1: The Fertility Factor

Two winters ago I traveled with my three daughters, Ari, Alex and Noa, and wife, Elise, to the snowy city of Cleveland to attend a Bar Mitzvah for a thirteen-year-old young man. A Bar Mitzvah, or Bat Mitzvah for a girl, is a traditional Jewish coming-of-age event in which family and friends gather for a five-century-old ceremony that includes the young person reading from the Old Testament. A reception is traditionally held after the service, and as we drove from the service to a downtown hotel for the reception on that cold, gray day, our daughters, ages seven, nine and eleven, bickered with each other as usual in the backseat.

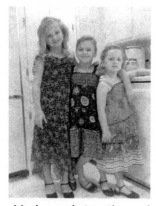

My three girls Ari, Alex and Noa all dressed and ready

Once at the hotel, we caught up with old friends, met new people, and enjoyed the warm party atmosphere of the typical Bar Mitzvah, including lots of kissing, hugging, loads of food, and maybe a drink or two. Most everyone wore the dark suits or black dresses commonly seen at that type of celebration and nobody expected anything out of the norm until . . . she walked in.

Everyone's eyes instantly went to her. She was a knockout—tall and fit in a sleek white dress that showed all her curves. Her striking appearance oozed sexiness and, even more important, confidence. She was hot and she knew it. It was no surprise that all the middle-aged, balding men were caught off guard and couldn't help but peek over their wives' shoulders and that thirteen-year-old boys cackled as they recognized inexplicable feelings surging in their bodies. As a scientist who studies first impressions, beauty and fertility, I understood all those reactions, but what caught me off guard was, Noa, my seven-year-old daughter's response. Too young to be stifled by the social norms that teach us to subdue our emotions and behaviors in public, she acted on her basic attractions. She didn't know anything about the concept of sexiness or mating or the power that a beautiful woman can have, but nonetheless, she was magnetized by this woman. For the rest of the night she was glued to her hip. We couldn't pull her away. I watched with academic curiosity and wondered why a little girl was so captivated by a strikingly beautiful thirty-year-old woman. Clearly this lady had something that tantalized not only the most primitive part of a male's brain but also that of a seven-year-old girl. My daughter helped me realize that the Fertility Factor is not necessarily sexual, but more commonly manifested as an undeniable attraction.

The Fertility Factor prompts a visceral reaction that compels us to reach out or back away.

Why Sugar is Sweet and
You're Not as Evolved as You Think

In order for our species to survive, human beings had to develop skills and aptitudes for finding food, building shelter and defending themselves. But our bodies were not designed to live in a society with grocery stores, life spans of eighty years, or static activities like watching television and sitting at desks for hours at a time.

Last summer five new shops opened up in my small suburban Chicago neighborhood selling ice cream, frozen yogurt, gelato, or muffins. Although most of the townspeople thought these stores were novel and trendy, most of us wondered how all five indulgent sweet shops would survive through the winter in our sparsely populated, health-conscious corner of the suburbs. As it turned out, they not only survived but thrived through that following winter with their doors open late every night. On the weekends there are still lines out the door. Why?

We all know far too well that sweets in excess are not healthy and that diabetes is a nutritional disease correlated with sugar intake, but every night my kids beg to go to one of the sweet shops. And once again it is a child's raw, uninhibited desires that help us better understand ourselves. Kids haven't yet learned to hamper those primitive cravings that we never outgrow. Every time I hear my daughters plead to go out for ice cream, I'm reminded of the wiring behind their love of sweets, a wiring we all share, young and old. Why are we so tantalized and driven to desire sweets in contrast to the other flavors that our taste buds recognize?

We've adapted to learn that foods that are firm with bright colors are energy packing, whereas soft foods with dark spots are diseased and spoiled. Our eyes have developed to find these foods and our tongues have evolved to like the taste of sweet foods. Why? Once again, it's all about survival. Sweet means sugar and our bodies can quickly digest and metabolize sugar, converting into a sudden boost of energy. This is critical if you are running away from a predator, on a mission to find your next meal or taking a long-distance trek. Because sweet foods are an excellent source of quick energy, our bodies developed to love sweet berries and figs; however, we have not yet evolved far enough to know when to turn off this desire. Living in a world with abundant sweets available at every turn, we are confronted with epidemics of obesity and diabetes, the nutrition-based diseases that were unlikely in the resource-sparse environment of our distant ancestors.

In the same way, we are wired with instinctual reactions to certain physical traits and cannot help making snap judgments about people. We are as programmed to respond to what we see in a person's face and body as we are to desire an energy-packed sugary snack.

The woman in white embodied the Fertility Factor, an undeniable aura that draws others in and is rooted in fertility. Her F1 Factor was also seasoned with firm confidence, and the combination created an irresistible attraction. Even on its own, however, the Fertility Factor doesn't discriminate. It attracts both genders and people of all ages. To this day my daughter, who is now nine years old, is incredibly attracted to those who exude beauty and confidence. I know my hands are full with this one—her newest prospect is Justin Bieber, whom she is convinced will be her husband one day.

We've all experienced the primal attraction of the Fertility Factor. Think back to the last time you were at a party and someone who walked into the room immediately captured your attention and maybe that of your best friend as well. Why? What did that person possess? Was he or she wearing especially fashionable clothing and a great smile, or was endowed with a knockout figure or physique? Did you desire to meet that person and learn his/her story, or were you intimidated, jealous and turned off? For most of us the Fertility Factor prompts a visceral reaction that compels us to reach out or back away. In the latter case, the encounter may bring up intimidating feelings based on our fear of rejection or a sense, also subconsciously, that the person doesn't fit the bill of the ideal man or woman. For those less hindered, the encounter could initiate a positive and rewarding experience.

> Since there is no escaping this primitive reflex, why not understand, control, and use it to your benefit?

Regardless of the outcome, we've all experienced these feelings and responses. In fact, we go through this scenario many times a week. It's human nature to constantly evaluate others and form initial judgments. Since there is no escaping this primitive reflex, why not understand, control, and use it to your benefit? We must keep in mind that at our core we are still animals. And although we now live in a "civilized" world, our needs and desires evolved and adapted from the harsh evolutionary environments of our ancient past. Most of our human struggles can be attributed to the never-ending conflicts that rage when our evolutionary instincts clash with the modern constructs of a society and civilization. The bottom line is—fertile people are appealing and we are hardwired to be attracted to them. You may like to think you are above such "shallow" behavior, but nature built in this response for the species' survival. It's as biologically critical as our positive response to something sweet.

> The bottom line is—fertile people are attractive and we are hardwired to be attracted to them.

Homo as a genus broke off the evolutionary tree about 4 million years ago and Homo sapiens around 250,000 year ago. It was only 50,000 years ago that we started to display culture and 10,000 years since we started to live in cities, or become civilized.

In other words—we've been civilized for less than 1% of our evolution as humans!

It's rather narcissistic to believe that our very recent cultural sophistication has dissolved the survival mechanisms that have evolved over millions of years, but maybe that shouldn't be so surprising. We like to put ourselves at the center of the universe. But only by letting go of our egos can we look at ourselves from a broad perspective and acknowledge that the human psyche is much more influenced by innate urges than by politics, religion, or laws. The most effective and easily followed rules of civilization are those that are consistent with our biological desires. The features of society that go against the natural grain give us problems and account for our struggles with high divorce rates, prostitution, and obesity. It's not easy to switch off the adaptive behaviors which have evolved over eons and are ingrained at the deepest level of our being to ensure survival.

All human beings are attracted to very similar things and evolutionary biology explains most of the reasons why. And perhaps the one thing we all want at least collectively more than anything else is immortality. Finding the ideal fertile mate is a critical step to achieving that timeless human desire.

The Smile of Immortality

After suffering a random seizure at age twenty-eight, my first cousin and best friend, Jeff, was diagnosed with a stage-three glioblastoma, a malignant brain tumor. His doctors told him he had ten years to live and that he could extend that by a few months if he could tolerate and undergo chemotherapy, which would make him lose all his hair and be sick throughout the treatment period. The doctors admitted that in rare cases the chemo was so toxic to the body that it could kill, but on the other hand, in some cases people had a complete remission of the tumor and became miracle patients. They also recommended that Jeff have MRI imaging studies of his brain taken twice a year to evaluate the size and progression of the tumor. Well, being contrarian and stubborn, Jeff decided against chemotherapy and the regular MRIs. He wanted to live the next ten years

> Perhaps the one thing we all want at least collectively, more than anything else is immortality, and finding the ideal fertile mate is a critical step to achieving it.

as if nothing was wrong, and that's what he began to do. He was committed to living life to the fullest.

After experimenting with every recreational drug he could get his hands on, traveling across the country with the Grateful Dead for a year, sleeping odd hours, and working as a DJ in a gentlemen's club, Jeff realized that he wanted one thing more than anything else—immortality. And instead of seeking out religion, he searched for a mate. He wanted a child. About five years into his illness Jeff met a beautiful woman, Aneba, who was working and attending school in Phoenix where he lived. Aneba was from Togo on the West Coast of Africa, and she and Jeff developed a meaningful relationship. Jeff told her that he wanted to have a child, but lacked the financial and emotional reserves to get married. He also mentioned that he had a disease, but Aneba didn't seem to be dissuaded by that or the criticisms that might fly their way by deciding to bring a life into the world that Jeff wouldn't be able to support. She understood why Jeff wanted to have a child, loved him and was willing to move ahead with the plan. They made it their secret and in early 2006 they had a beautiful young girl, Rianna.

> From the perspective of an evolutionary biologist, human beings have only one purpose on earth—to procreate and forge a more genetically fit species.

As they expected, some of the people in their lives turned their decision into a controversy. How could he do this? Who is going to pay for the baby after he's gone? Who will be the father? But Jeff would hear nothing of it. He doted on his baby girl and was deeply fulfilled. Unfortunately, Jeff and Aneba's relationship faded and a couple years later Jeff's condition took a turn for the worse. He and Aneba had split up and Jeff had to be content with phoning his daughter from time to time. He couldn't talk because the tumor had affected the speech centers in his brain, so he listened to her on the phone and smiled from ear to ear when he heard her voice. Sadly, Jeff passed away the following year. Aneba and the baby went back to Africa and there was a lot of disappointment in Jeff's family at the prospect of not seeing them anymore. However, Aneba had other ideas. She insisted that the baby have a relationship with her biological aunts, uncles, cousins, and grandmother, even if only by keeping in touch over the phone.

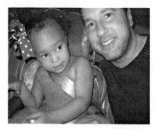

Jeff and his daughter Rianna.

Two years later Aneba remarried a wonderful man, they moved to Arizona and went on to have more children. Her new husband adopted Rianna, but they both agreed that the girl should know and feel connected to her biological roots. We were thrilled that they sent Rianna to Chicago for a two-week visit over the holidays in 2011. To our family's delight, young Rianna looks every bit like my cousin Jeff. She resembles him physically and walks, talks, and smiles just like him. My family couldn't be happier because Jeff is still alive in her. And I can't help thinking that Jeff knew exactly what he was doing. He found immortality by leaving a legacy in the form of his genes.

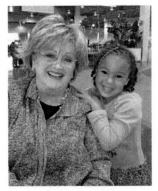

Rianna and her grandmother, my Aunt Judy.

There is an evolutionary explanation why most religions have defined an afterlife or heaven. Our need to believe that we don't just die and leave this earth is based on a well-established biological law: beneath the spiritual hope is an animalistic and primitive desire for the immortality of our genes. The idea of the immortal soul may be one of humanity's translations of that biological desire. From the perspective of an evolutionary biologist, human beings have only one purpose on earth, and that is to procreate and forge a more genetically fit species. Protecting your genes by finding the perfect, fertile mate who will nurture your offspring until they live to a self-supportive age assures that your genes will survive to the next generation. For those who cannot or do not desire having their own children, likely still feel an urge to protect and nurture closely related nieces, nephews and cousins. In biological terms a motivation to project our genetic lineage ahead drives most every one of us. And in order to find the ideal mate to fulfill that drive we must have a sharp sense of who is healthy and fertile. That's why Mother Nature or the higher being that created us designed physical signs of fertility to be attractive.

F2: The Fear Factor

First impressions evolved to help ensure our genetic immortality through every critical phase of our lives. After delivering a baby into the world that carries our genetic material it is critical we protect it until it can fend for itself. From a primitive perspective, children become self-sufficient somewhere around the age of seven when they are able to gather their own food and are no longer reliant on their mother for transportation or breast-feeding. And while in modern times its normal for children to live at home with their parents well past the age of eighteen, seven years still represents a critical age in our society. Studies show that the odds of a couple breaking up are highest when their first child reaches the age of seven (Morgan, Lye &Condran, 1988).

> The shorter life span of our primitive ancestors may explain the "seven-year itch."

This may explain the "seven-year itch."

An alert seems to buzz inside, warning that it's time to have another child or move on to a more fertile mate.

Our bodies have not caught up with the fact that we live much longer. Until relatively recently, human life expectancy was only in the late thirties or early forties, so we had to quickly get on with the business of living and become self-reliant sooner rather than later.

In a primitive existence, fathers were likely off on a hunt for days at a time with other tribesmen looking for food. Mothers had to feed the children and keep them and the dwelling safe. At an early age, children may have wandered off a bit looking for berries or something else to eat. What if a lion, hyena, or hungry alligator spotted them? A child would quickly have to learn to recognize that big teeth, growling, and threatening postures all indicate that an animal was a threat to its existence. As a result, the ability to detect danger is perhaps the most quickly processed and primitive neural pathway in our brain (Cosmides&Tooby, 1994). If our species wasn't able to quickly detect and assess danger, we wouldn't be able to reach sexual maturation and pass on our genes.

> The ability to detect danger is perhaps the most quickly processed and primitive neural pathway in our brain.

When we perceive a threat, primitive neural pathways in the amygdala and cingulate cortex of the brain are stimulated to elicit an immediate response. It is a visceral sense that kicks in automatically. How many times have you sensed that something was wrong, even though you didn't see any overt signs of danger? You weren't sure why, but you just knew a threat was nearby. This is the gut response that tells you to get out of there, and fast. Why are movies like *Halloween* and *The Sixth Sense* so captivating? World-class directors have mastered the art of teasing the Fear Factor.

The deeply imbedded response within the Fear Factor is ignited by specific physical features and cues that the brain perceives as threatening. When we see a man with heavyset brows, an overly broad jaw, or darkly contrasted, close-set eyes, our brain instantly processes those features and sends up a red flag. Hollywood horror movies play up these features in characters like Frankenstein, Dracula and the Wolfman because we're hard-wired to get a jolt of fear from just one glance.

In fact, we know that these physical traits are indeed signals of more aggressive men. Threatening-looking facial structures go hand in hand with an excess of testosterone during development stages, and studies prove that men with these higher levels are more aggressive, dominant, unfriendly, controlling, manipulative, selfish and potentially more likely to be convicted of committing crimes. While there are many other factors associated with criminality, high levels of testosterone are found in single males and males in competitive situations. In one study from Canada that linked facial appearance to aggressive behaviors, subjects looking at neutral photos of college and professional hockey players matched dominant facial appearance to aggressive behaviors. The subjects singled out men with wide jaws as more aggressive, for example, and those choices were accurate because the wide-jawed men had racked up more penalty minutes on the rink (Carré& McCormick, 2008). No wonder, then, that

> Men with excess testosterone are more aggressive, dominant, unfriendly, controlling, manipulative and selfish.

over millions of years nature has taught women to fear men with these features. Women rely on stable relationships for their offspring to survive, and pairing up with an overly aggressive man could be too risky.

We don't want to base our entire impression of someone on a few facial features alone, of course. Judging people along those lines has led to some of the world's worst atrocities. As a matter of fact, as we continue to evolve, our higher intellect is adapting because it is learning that our intuition isn't always perfect. We have all backtracked on a judgment or two we made about someone based on a first impression, and our survival responses are still a work in progress. We can't dismiss, however, that our brains have evolved over hundreds of thousands of years to instantly recognize a threat. And I mean *instantly*.

In a Princeton University study about the timing of our impressions, subjects looked at photos of actors for a fraction of a second and were asked to judge these people based on appearance alone. Their answers were compared to those of others looking at the photo without any time limit. The impression made within 100 milliseconds (a tenth of a second) was virtually the same as that made after a longer look (Willis &Todorov, 2006). This shows that our split-second powers of perception are as reliable as the more lengthy inspections we make of others. Another amazing fact uncovered in this study involves our ability to recognize if someone is trustworthy or

> Nature puts the highest priority on making sure we can instantly size up whether someone is harmless or a threat.

not. The subjects gauged trustworthiness more efficiently than any other trait, revealing that nature puts the highest priority on making sure we can instantly size up whether someone is harmless or a threat.

We are also hard-wired to view babies as non-threatening and feel caring and affectionate toward them. Our brains have evolved to trigger a protective and nurturing response when we see baby-like characteristics such as a large head and big eyes— from baby dolphins and calves to human infants, we can't help but feel affection for the innocent. This attraction runs deep and affects us physically: a woman's pupils will dilate—an attraction response—when she looks at a baby.

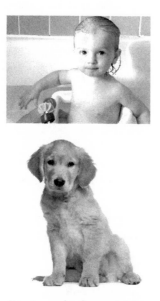

Puppies and infants with large, wide, non-threatening eyes

While horror filmmakers play on our subconscious fears of dark brows and big jaws, cartoonists and advertisers draw on our innate affection for infants. Disney® animators capitalize on this by giving their characters large eyes, small chins, light skin, and other infantile features. We're programmed to gaze affectionately and want to protect Snow White, Tinker Bell, and the Little Mermaid. Ad makers appeal to our primitive drives by putting babies in commercials for tires (we want to protect them with the best) and online trading services—who can resist babies acting smart and tech-savvy? Marketers are shrewd students of human nature.

Women can take advantage of our natural, instinctual attraction and affection for those with infantile features by enhancing them in themselves. Even the subtlest changes in this direction can have an enormously positive effect on the first impression a woman projects.

From clothing and hairstyles to makeup and cosmetic treatments, we can consciously alter, accentuate, or deemphasize the "F" Factors that contribute to how we are perceived by others at first glance. If we want to improve our chances of making a positive first impression and reap all the benefits that come with it, we must take a close look at the signals we're putting out.

Do your signals add up to an irresistible force of attraction?

The physical characteristics of raw beauty that we are prewired to recognize such as symmetry and an ideal waist-to-hip ratio are not the only factors of attraction—

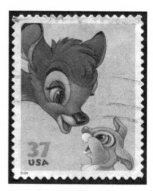

Disney characters with large eyes.

far from it. Signals that come from less obvious traits such as expression, self-esteem, posture, clothing, odor, hairstyle, adornments and cosmetics can outdo those factors and produce a striking first impression and attractiveness.

The physical characteristics of raw beauty that we are prewired to recognize are not the only factors of attraction—far from it.

While we have little control over our raw beauty, we have some control over our attractiveness and almost complete control over the impression we project. This is why a masculine hunk can be

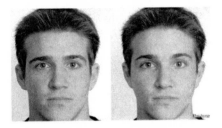

In a study about masculine features and male attractiveness, photographs were digitally altered to show variations on male features: at left, the more "manly" face is wider, while the face at the right has been adjusted for a smaller chin and larger eyes, two features associated with youthful innocence. (Image: Economist, 2010)

considered the sexiest man alive one day and a vulgar idiot the next, and a young star's reputation as a beauty icon switched overnight into that of a tramp. In all walks of life, the skill and mastery of crafting the first impression often makes the difference between success and failure.

CHAPTER 2

THE SEXIEST RACIST ALIVE

I n 1985 actor Mel Gibson was one of the hottest actors in Hollywood. He had starred in three Mad Max movies and received critical acclaim for his roles in *The Year of Living Dangerously* and *Gallipoli*. The film critic Vincent Canby remarked, "I can't define 'star quality,' but whatever it is, Mr. Gibson has it." *People* magazine anointed him the heartthrob of the nation by selecting him for the cover of the very first Sexiest Man Alive issue. Gibson was not only a sex symbol, but also a respected family man who brought his wife and seven children with him from Australia to the United States. His career continued to thrive through the 1990s, culminating with *Braveheart*, which won five Oscars including Best Picture and Best Director.

It seemed nothing could derail this hunk—until the mid-2000s, when a few cracks began to show in Gibson's veneer. It started with *The Passion of the Christ*, the controversial movie he co–wrote, produced, and directed in 2004. While some critics admired the film's artistic expression, others thought it was anti-Semitic and historically inaccurate. In spite of the mixed response, the movie was a commercial success with box office receipts grossing over 300 million dollars. Evidence of Gibson's cultural insensitivity intensified when the Gay Lesbian Alliance Against Defamation (GLADD) accused him of homophobia based on derogatory comments he had made against homosexuals.

But the hidden side of Gibson's personality broke out in full force when he was stopped for drunk driving in July 2006. Police caught him speeding with open liquor in his car and the drunken tirade of ethnic slurs that exploded from him during the arrest—"F---ing Jews, the Jews are responsible for all the wars in the

> Our perceptions of beauty and attractiveness can be worlds apart.

world"—made headline news. His star status took a beating when his mug shot was pasted all over TV and the Internet. He pleaded no contest to misdemeanor drunk driving charges and was sentenced to three years of probation. But four years later his

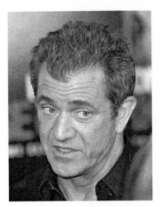

Angry Mel

superstar image probably took its greatest tumble when he was taped yelling angry profanities at his girlfriend, Oksana Grigorieva, the mother of two of his children. His vulgar outrage, which was broadcast all over the media, resulted in a restraining order and domestic violence investigation. Soon afterward the William Morris Agency dropped him and in March 2011 he pleaded no contest to a misdemeanor battery charge.

Gibson is still handsome today, but his Hollywood image has been scarred by his six-year run showing the world his absolute worst side.

And Mel is not the only star who can make pretty look ugly.

Actress, model and pop singer Lindsay Lohan broke onto the scene in the 1998 hit remake of *The Parent Trap*, which earned her a best performance award from the Youth in Film Awards, known as the "Kiddie Oscars." Her next film, *Freaky Friday*, won her the Breakthrough Performance Award at the 2004 MTV Awards, and her role in *Mean Girls* the following year cemented her success. Critics admired her, young girls idolized her, and teen boys fantasized about her, but in 2007 her image took a serious blow. After being convicted of driving under the influence and cocaine possession for the second time, she was sentenced to one day in prison and ten days of community

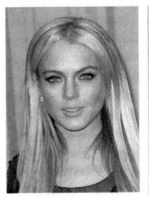
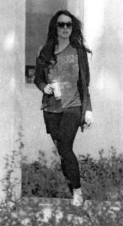

Lindsay Lohan was once an idol for teenage females and males alike.

service. But instead of stopping or slowing down her criminal behavior, she got even more reckless and launched a string of crimes that led to more convictions and prison and rehab time. Her mug shot went viral and she became the butt of many late-night TV jokes. The attractive pinup who once posed naked for a *Playboy* spread is now more known for her look in prison oranges. Lindsay went from teenage princess to strung-out drug queen in the same amount of time most kids start and finish high school. Or as my daughter, Ari, likes to describe her, "She is iconic because she is ironic."

We all know people who are physically gorgeous but appear highly unattractive. Our perceptions of beauty and attractiveness can be worlds apart. It all depends on what's going on with the sender and receiver.

Beauty is a Game of Catch

In baseball, how a pitcher throws a ball determines where and how the catcher is supposed to catch it. The ball is analogous to beauty, and how that beauty is thrown or projected determines whether the observer finds it attractive or not. Beauty is limited by both the way it is delivered and the manner in which it is perceived. Beauty, no matter how stunning, can be completely overlooked if the catcher isn't ready to receive it.

> Beauty, no matter how stunning, can be completely overlooked if the catcher isn't ready to receive it.

During morning rush hour on January 12, 2007, the famed violinist Joshua Bell stood at the entrance to a Metro station in downtown Washington, D.C., and played one classical masterpiece after another. Of the more than one thousand people who passed by, only seven stopped for a brief minute to listen. The hurried pedestrians barely noticed that one of the world's most acclaimed musicians, playing on a multi-million-dollar Stradivarius violin, was giving them what sold-out audiences all over the world clamored after. Only three days earlier Bell had performed at Boston Symphony Hall, where the mediocre seats went for a hundred dollars apiece. After forty-five minutes of a masterful performance in the subway entrance, his violin case had only thirty-two dollars to show for it.

The Washington Post conducted this social experiment in attempt to see if Joshua Bell's beautiful music could be perceived in a different environment. The crowds' lack of interest proved that the manner in which his artistry was presented was as critical to how it would be appreciated and perceived, if not more so, than the inherent beauty of the music itself. This combination of raw beauty and the delivery system in which it's transferred and perceived is the defining structure of the first impression.

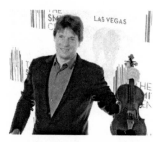

Josh Bell, famed violinist who made beautiful music in a subway and orchestra hall

Like a scanner, our brain is constantly absorbing impressions of people and interpreting and acting on those perceptions. Developed for species survival, the first impression is critical to us on a personal level.

First Impressions and Your Potential Mate

Once your perceptions have protected you long enough to get you to sexual maturity, the second and most important role of first impressions zones in on helping you find a mate. First impressions bridge the gap from beauty to attraction. When the signals push all the right buttons in the receiver, the brain draws out the most primitive subconscious form of communication—raw, animalistic passion. But this is the twenty-first century, not the Pleistocene, so falling prey to our primitive first impressions can be misleading. The strapping hunk that your instincts tell you is a good provider could actually be a dead-broke dropout living in his mom's basement. On the other hand, you may be the one unknowingly projecting a first impression that doesn't accurately reflect all your strengths and fine qualities. Either way, understanding how first impressions transform simple beauty into passionate attraction gives an invaluable edge.

> When the signals push all the right buttons in the receiver, the brain draws out the most primitive subconscious form of communication— raw, animalistic passion.

Beauty, impressions, attraction . . . how can such intimately related parts of human experience be so separate and unique? To put each in its rightful place, let's think of appearances as a language. Just as some languages sound more beautiful than others, some appearances are more beautiful than others. Much of the beauty of language is conveyed through the tone, tempo and rhythm of the speaker. Similarly, we perceive much of the beauty of someone's appearance through a combination of subconscious observations of symmetry, bone structure, poise and expression in a manifestation called the impression. This impression then leads to the all-important concept of attractiveness. However, without all the other elements that go into the impression, beauty is simply something that exists in isolation and is either unrecognized or under-appreciated.

Defining Beauty

The meaning of beauty has been debated for millennia. The ancient Greek poet Sappho associated it with personal goodness, writing, "What is beautiful is good, and who is good will soon be beautiful." About a century later, Plato defined beauty as one of the unchanging "Forms" that make up the higher, invisible reality that exists above the physical world. According to his philosophy, we recognize objects as beautiful because they are associated with the eternal Form of Beauty. The eighteenth-century philosopher Immanuel Kant believed beauty is that which evokes a universal rather than merely personal pleasure.

Confucius observed that beauty is in the eye of the beholder: "Everything has its beauty, but not everyone sees it."

You're probably familiar with dozens of other descriptions of beauty, too, but you may not have heard it defined like this:

Beauty, in its purest essence, is a form of subconscious communication between two individuals. It is the body's way of saying, "I am healthy, well, and fertile." In nature's eyes, beauty is a form of subliminal communication designed to describe our genes.

As a scientist, I look to Charles Darwin for this practical view of beauty. According to the process of natural selection, beauty is a tool for ensuring the survival of our genes. Nancy Etcoff's groundbreaking book on beauty, which I highly recommend, discusses scientific evaluations, history, and anecdotes to pull together her own eclectic definition (Etcoff, 2000). In the rawest sense of physical beauty, we have come to associate certain physical traits such as facial and bodily symmetry, averageness, specific body-size ratios and youthfulness with beauty. We will delve into these characteristics in later chapters, but first we'll take a broader look at beauty from an evolutionary perspective.

> The value nature puts on beauty is every bit as important to our survival as the value put on our sweet sense of taste.

To appreciate beauty is to recognize that the value nature puts on beauty is every bit as important to our survival as the value put on our ability to taste sweets. Over millions of years, humans have developed genetic codes for physical traits that have helped us overcome threats to our species. The environment throws us many curve balls and human beings have to either adapt to them or die off.

How does nature select traits that are considered beautiful and push them along to keep the species going? The story of another genetic trait, the sickle cell, gives us a simple straightforward example of how adaptation takes place.

Sickle cell disease reveals how genes that are beneficial to human survival proliferate in a culture. As the most common inherited blood disorder in the United States, sickle cell disease affects about 70,000 people. One in 500 African Americans has the disease and eight percent of African Americans carry the gene. Those who suffer from the disease experience painful cramping episodes, infection, blood vessel obstruction, stroke, and even death.

> To celebrate the superiority of their fit genetic makeup, people develop external clues to tell the world how great their genes are. We identify those clues as beauty.

However, in certain parts of the world, specifically the Mediterranean and the West Coast of Africa, sickle cells are an adaptive trait allowing one to survive in the presence of malaria. Malaria is caused by a blood-borne parasite called *Plasmodium falciparum* that is carried by mosquitoes and gets into the bloodstream through a mosquito bite. Those who carry one of the sickle cell genes develop red blood cells that have a slightly different shape, one in which the parasite cannot survive. These individuals avoid the deadly disease, thrive and pass on their sickle gene to their offspring. Those sickle cell individuals then pass on their malaria-resistant gene to their children and so on throughout the generations.

In the process of natural selection, a genetic alteration that is beneficial to an individual is more likely to be passed on to the next generation. This individual survives and passes it on to more people until the new genetic type (genotype) and its intended physical manifestation (phenotype) spreads throughout the community, allowing a species to survive past a threat. When this happens, we say the genetic change is "adaptive."

In a very similar manner, the physical manifestation, or phenotype, of beauty is adaptive to our species and critical to our survival. People who are genetically heterozygous (varied) likely possess a better, fit genetic sequence (genotype). And to celebrate this superiority, individuals develop external clues (phenotypes) to tell the world about their great genes. Over time, we learn to identify and associate these external clues as beauty.

You can debate the meaning of beauty with philosophers and poets as much as you want, but as far as nature is concerned, it's the best tool in the box to keep not only the human species moving forward but all of nature. It is perhaps the rawest of all energies fueling evolution.

Defining Attractiveness

We now see that beauty is the universal language of health. But how that message is projected is another matter. The impression we project is the dialect, tempo, and tone of beauty's language. Just like a magnificent poem can be crudely delivered or the French language spoiled by a strong American accent, a beautiful person may project an impression that is interpreted as unattractive. The opposite is also true: a person who is physically less than beautiful may appear highly attractive by presenting him- or herself in a favorable way. Being born beautiful may be a gift, but being able to present oneself in an attractive manner is even more powerful.

> Being born beautiful may be a gift, but being able to present oneself in an attractive manner is even more powerful.

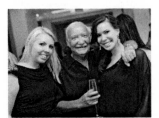
My charming dad

My father is not what you would traditionally call the most attractive man. He stands at about five-foot-six, wears large glasses and a mustache, is bald with a few fine gray hairs combed over the top, has a turkey neck and deeply etched wrinkles, and talks with a foreign accent. But wow—can he charm the pants off anyone.

When Dad walks into a room, he captures everyone's attention. He fears nothing and no one. He will approach the most beautiful woman or most intimidating man and strike up a conversation. My father thinks he is the best-looking man in the room. He has enormous self-confidence and everyone in the room perceives it.

Such robust self-confidence is highly attractive.

An example from my practice proves the same point. Recently, a thirty-two-year-old woman came in to see me to have her nose fixed; it was one of the most unattractive, broken, and misshapen noses I have ever seen. Additionally, she had crooked yellow teeth, a heavy figure, and small beady eyes. Yet she exuded so much confidence. She had a powerful job, her boyfriend was a TV personality, and she flipped her hair as if she was a beauty queen. She thought she was beautiful, and because of this, she gave an impression that she was, which in turn was felt by my staff and everyone else who met her.

On the other hand, I often see both men and women who are physically gorgeous, possessing all the ideal angles and facial contours characteristic of ideal beauty, but they don't seem to project it. They walk in with their head low, slumped over and appear very introverted as they shuffle in. While they are physically beautiful, their projected personalities do not reveal beauty; they lack attractiveness.

Attractiveness is a fluid, abstract impression formulated by the basic elements of beauty. However, being perceived attractive is more than just possessing the raw chemical compositions of beauty. Attractiveness is dynamic, relative to the social and cultural norms of the times along with the moment-by-moment motivation of the observer. Attractiveness requires the active, yet subconscious, participation of the observer to interpret the projected impression. Our ability to interpret beauty as attractiveness is rooted in all the accumulated and inherited information in our conscious and subconscious mind, which has been acquired through culture, previous experiences and our evolutionary instincts.

Other factors that influence the impression you make include posture, odor, clothing and facial expression— all of which can be developed and strengthened to your great advantage.

Without impressions there is no attraction. Beauty is more likely to be perceived as attractive when it's delivered and accepted in the appropriate way. Joshua Bell gave those commuters a world-class performance, but he delivered it in the unfitting context of a metro station. The beauty didn't have a chance.

Delivery is crucial to how an impression is interpreted, as is the state of mind of the observer. If a physically beautiful person brushes past you the day you are grieving a loss, you may not recognize that person as attractive. However, six months later, while on vacation in Hawaii, that same person may bump into you while you're relaxing at the Tiki bar and command every ounce of your attention.

Changing cultural norms also impact how we perceive a person's impression. Today, many consider smoking unattractive and the smell or appearance of a cigarette can morph a physically beautiful person into a repulsive one. A couple of generations ago, however, Humphrey Bogart or Lauren Bacall seemed to ooze sexiness while lounging with a cigarette hanging from their lower lip. In the sixteenth century, Queen Elizabeth, the Virgin Queen, painted her face ivory white to mimic the flawless skin of youth, but by today's Western standards that overblown effect would give the impression of sickliness or anemia. However, if you lived in Tokyo you would see the faces of twenty-first century Geishas donning that pale appearance, attempting to project a youthful impression.

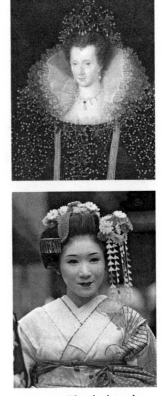

Queen Elizabeth and a Geisha, both with porcelain-colored skin

Attraction Beyond Beauty

All of the above reveals that raw beauty is not the last word in attractiveness. Other factors that influence the impression include posture, odor, clothing and facial expression—all of which can be developed and strengthened to an advantage. Posture, for example, speaks volumes.

In a meaningful study published in 2009, photographs were taken of 123 undergraduate students. First, they were asked to pose with a neutral expressions and stances (Naumann, Vazire, Rentfrow& Gosling, 2009). Then they were allowed to stand in a relaxed, natural pose. Observers were asked to rate their personalities in ten categories (extroversion, agreeability, conscientiousness, emotional stability, openness, likability, self-esteem, loneliness, religiosity and political orientation). Whether the students were asked to pose stoically or in a natural relaxed posture, observers could accurately determine which ones were most extroverted. Self-esteem was also easily identified.

Observers could also detect qualities of openness and likability. This confirms that how we stand and carry ourselves not only affects first impressions, but also gives non-verbal clues about key elements of our personality. Good posture broadcasts openness and confidence. It's a subtle physical cue that shows the world you are ready

Good posture broadcasts openness and confidence— and is very attractive.

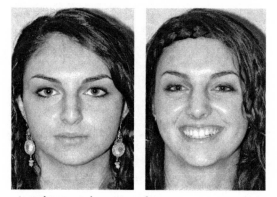

A smile can make a pretty face even more attractive.

to handle whatever comes your way. *It's very attractive.*

A pleasant smell can make a rather plain person seem more attractive and a bad smell can quickly make a beautiful person unappealing. A heavy brow, angry scowl and deep vertical creases between the eyebrows are perceived in a negative way, but a big smile projects a friendly, successful impression. In a study we did in 2008, over 300 unknowing observers were asked to record their first impressions of photographed headshots of random people (Dayan, Lieberman, Thakkar, Larimer & Anstead, 2008). The images of the person smiling were perceived to be more attractive, successful at dating, athletic, and academically superior than those images without a smile.

Confidence, First Impressions, and Attractiveness

As a plastic surgeon, I believe my goal is to make people feel more confident in their appearance. Many people view plastic surgeons as purveyors of beauty for the vanity-challenged, and while my profession in part bears the burden of fault, it is my belief that nothing could be further from the truth. Plastic surgeons possess the skills, talent and tools to make people more physically beautiful, but this may not help them feel more confident or improve their self-esteem.

And there is no benefit to looking more beautiful if one doesn't feel more beautiful.

Self-esteem is the essential ingredient I can provide in my practice. People with a lot of confidence exude it in their expression, posture, and aura. I recently treated a high school senior who wanted a nose job (rhinoplasty). Ryan was deeply bothered by his nose but afraid to tell his single, hard-working mom that he wanted to do something about it. They were a family of modest means and his mother was working long hours to support her only son who was clearly her pride and joy. He came into my office with his hands in his pockets and a slouch that allowed his shaggy hair to cover his acne-ridden face. His blue jeans hung off his hips and his shoelaces trailed behind his dragging feet.

Ryan was ashamed to tell his mom that he wanted surgery and was sure she wouldn't be able to afford it. But his eyes lit up when I showed him, via computer simulation, what he could look like with a different nose. His mom recognized the desire in her son and together we put a plan in place to make his rhinoplasty a reality. The surgery went well and soon afterward an email came across my desk from Ryan's mom that she sent to my patient coordinator, Katie. Here's part of that message:

"Ryan looks wonderful and I can see the self-confidence growing every day. This was the best decision we could have made. I am so glad I found a way, because when Ryan looked at himself in the mirror the day the splint was taken off, there is no price that could be put on the expression on his face. This procedure has already changed Ryan's life for the better, and in turn has changed mine, too. Thank you so very much from the bottom of our hearts."

If you inherited the characteristics of what nature defines as physical beauty, they are only as beneficial as far as they are delivered. The *impression* created is more important in terms of gaining an advantage in all personal and professional relationships. And the secret to enhancing that impression boils down to one word: confidence.

Confidence is the key ingredient to appearing attractive. It is what allows you to feel beautiful in a brand-new dress or a new suit. When you show up at an event you want to feel good. If the morning of that event you feel thick and bloated and put yourself down for it, it doesn't matter how gorgeous that new dress is. If you don't feel confident, the dress alone isn't going to make a great impression. In science, we call that confidence self-esteem, and everything I've learned and witnessed convinces me that self-esteem is the essential ingredient to appearing more attractive and ultimately achieving greater success and satisfaction in life.

> The impression you create is more important than physical beauty, and the secret to enhancing that impression boils down to one word: confidence.

Those who think they are more attractive believe they deserve a more attractive mate and will not settle for less. The authors of a 2008 study wanted to determine the importance of objective physical attractiveness and compared it to the impact of one's own perception of attractiveness (Montoya, 2008). They found that the level of attractiveness people perceive of themselves, rooted in their self-esteem, is a highly significant factor in whom they choose to date and pursue. If we think we're attractive, then we're much less likely to fear rejection from a highly attractive person.

Not long ago, one of my patients exclaimed during a consultation, "Doctor, please help me. Everyone is staring at this horrible mark on my face. It's destroying me—everyone sees it!" She looked at me as if I could easily see her damaging mark. I could not help but notice the jagged, three-inch scar running vertically along her right cheek, but rather than point it out I asked, "Which mark are you referring to?" She then pointed to a tiny, barely-visible red spider vein on the left side of her forehead and said, "The red blemish, can't you see it? It makes me look so ugly and it's driving me crazy." She was not at all concerned with the rather large scar carved into her cheek, which I later learned was caused by an injury when she was two years old. She had adapted to it years ago and it did not affect her perception of her beauty. I deleted the red dot on her forehead and she walked out my door feeling prettier and walking taller.

Confidence 101

I have three daughters and it always amazes me how different they are, regardless of how similar they look. My youngest, Noa, even at nine years old, is filled with confidence and thinks she can achieve whatever she puts her mind to. She is always the first to volunteer and wants to be in the front of the line. She fears nothing, it seems, and I often have to smooth out her rough bravado in order to avoid offending others. If I can teach her how to channel her invincible confidence to do good for others, I will be satisfied. The other day she was telling me how she is the leader at school and all the other girls follow her. I asked her if she was nice to all the kids and she said, "Yes, but Dad, do you mean the weird ones, too?" Argh…I have a lot of work to do with this one.

> Everyone has the power to boost their confidence, or self-esteem, and reap all the rewards of making a dynamic and positive first impression.

My other daughters need a bit more encouragement before taking on a new task and are more sensitive about how their actions affect others. As much as I believe birth order has some influence on behavior, I also think these kids are just prewired differently. My youngest just happens to have the extra confidence gene. But I also believe that confidence can be cultivated and organically developed, and that it responds to encouragement.

We've all experienced the shot of positive energy that comes from getting a little praise. All of a sudden we walk

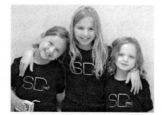

My three girls

taller, become the life of the party, and start attracting people. Similarly, one negative comment can quickly destroy our confidence, making us shy away and even want to leave the party. In one confidence study, men were asked to judge female attractiveness based on a phone call and subsequently being shown photos intended to represent the woman on the other end of the line (Zuckerman & Driver, 1989). When the photo was of a very attractive woman, the men's voices changed to one of being more endearing. Even more interesting the women, in response to the men's heightened voices, also became vocally more engaging and their physical actions more animated. They responded positively to the male's voice, showing increased confidence in their behavior.

Conversely, false confidence and cockiness are unattractive because we subconsciously detect them as deceitful. Just as seasoning can't overcome the bad taste of spoiled food, false bravado can't adequately hide a weakness in character. Human perception is almost always dead on—we intuitively know that excess cockiness is a cover-up. However, we are wired to respond positively to genuine confidence and find it attractive. We respect confidence in our greatest leaders and reject false assuredness or cockiness in others.

> As much as seventy percent of our self-esteem is based on our perception of our physical appearance.

While we do see an increase in overall confidence and self-esteem as we age, as much as seventy percent of our self-esteem is based on our perception of our physical appearance (Baumeister, Campbell, Krueger &Vohs, 2003). We begin to recognize the effects of appearance at an early age and start to understand where we fall in the spectrum of beauty. This is one reason young adolescents and teenagers spend so much time looking in the mirror and why I see many teenagers come to my office seeking nasal reshaping. And yes, we're influenced by our parents, family, and the peer environment in which we're raised, but we all possess the ability to alter our future. As we age, there seems to be greater insight and appreciation into our body's abilities and we seem to become less dissatisfied with our appearance, even if we gain weight (Garner, 1997).

Many who achieve professional success gain confidence that can be translated into all other aspects of their lives. No matter where our confidence comes from, it will translate into projecting a more attractive impression in both our professional and personal lives. On the other hand, if we lose confidence, we may shatter our attractive impression. The high school senior who at eighteen years old was voted the "best looking" in class may not feel the same way at her

> Identifying what enhances your confidence/self-esteem—and making time to integrate those activities into your life—is the best investment of time you'll ever make.

ten-year reunion if she is leading a life below her expectations, and her diminished attractiveness will show it.

The shortest route to projecting an attractive impression is to cultivate and invest in self-confidence, and this can be done in many ways. We all know the story of the awkward high school loner who didn't seem to care much for his appearance, stayed in and studied all the time and was teased by the popular kids, only to show up at the twenty-year reunion a millionaire with all the confidence in the world. He's dressed to the nines and has a well-defined figure and youthful, energetic gleam in his eye that makes everyone gravitate to him. How did that happen?

Some people gain confidence through athletic, personal, or professional achievement, while others practice meditation. Some use cosmetics and fashions while others take prescribed medication or undergo therapy to treat the aspects of their personality that are holding them back. One path does not mutually exclude another, and the gain in confidence has a dramatic effect on our appearance and the impression we project.

If self-confidence is the key to a positive first impression, a thoughtful and strategized route for evaluating oneself is essential for building confidence. This is the most difficult hurdle. An honest, candid and perhaps uncomfortable assessment of what truly depletes or enhances one's self-esteem as viewed through a naked lens can be incredibly beneficial. It then allows a schedule to be arranged devoid of self-defeating undertakings and filled with confidence enhancing activities.

An exercise I do with my class

Consider looking into a mirror, standing straight and tall, intently and purposefully staring into your own eyes. Asking yourself... who you are, what do you want and why do you want it. If you're honest with yourself, and you will know if you are, no matter what the answer maybe, this exercise could turn out to be one of the best investments of time and focus you'll ever make.

CHAPTER 3

CAUTION:
CURVES AHEAD!

"Disney heroines are *always* beautiful, shapely, and often sexually attractive."
—From *Understanding Disney* by Janet Wasko

Nobody knows how to exploit the most stereotypical traits of beauty like Disney. Large eyes and lips, small noses and chins, narrow waists and long hair— Disney's female characters flaunt these overemphasized qualities in every film and storybook. The plots are idealized, too; the princess always seems to get her prince and is rewarded for her beauty and righteousness. In contrast, bad girls like Maleficent, the Evil Queen, and Ursula are as unattractive as their nasty ways. Appearance and behavior are inextricably linked.

When my wife and I took our three girls to Disney World, I thought they would be excited about the rides, but all they wanted to do was meet and have breakfast, lunch, and dinner with the princesses in their castles. They each had their favorite and were sure to wear that one's dress as they scoured the park for their heroines. When they found their match, their eyes shot wide open and mouths dropped in awe. And they weren't the only ones. Lines of young girls stood beside them, whipped into a frenzy about meeting the

princess of their dreams. Even the adults looked excited
and intrigued by the Disney royalty.

These characters tap into something deep in
the human psyche, a visceral, unconscious force that
is part of our imprinting. Young and old respond to
their beauty with the same satisfying emotions that get
stirred up by the smells that bring back happy memories
from childhood such as crayons, Play Doh or cooking
reminiscent of our grandmother's kitchen. Beauty, like
a wonderful smell, stamps a favorable memory into
our brains, and the Disney studios know this very
well. From *Snow White* of 1937 to *Tangled* of 2010,
Disney is the master of redressing old, familiar tales
with an emphasis on exaggerated features of beauty
that electrify our innate, prewired senses.

Beauty Speaks to Us All

In the scientific world, beauty is raw, definable, and
utilitarian. It serves a purpose. Evolutionary biologists
look at beauty as a feature that nature favors in evolution
because it is an external indication of health, vitality, and
good genes. As a result, our ability to recognize these
tenets of beauty is prewired and innate. Some, like
Naomi Wolf, the noted feminist scholar and author,
argue that the standards of beauty are media-driven
by men on Madison Avenue in a deliberate attempt to
subjugate females (*The Beauty Myth*); however, science
seems to refute this. Infants as young as three months

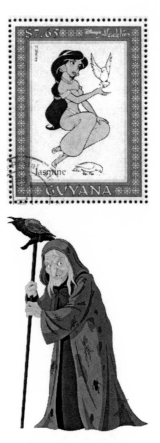

*Disney knows how to
characterize beauty and
unattractiveness better
than anyone else.*

old can recognize beautiful faces and stare at them longer than less beautiful ones
(Slater et al., 1998).

Other studies also confirm that the language of beauty is universal and engrained in
our species.

Researchers who spent years in the field studying remote and native Indian tribes
of Venezuela and Paraguay learned that these individuals who had little to no exposure
to TV, movies or magazines were as attracted to the same facial characteristics as
observers from Brazil, the United States, and Russia, despite little or no exposure to
Western media (Jones & Hill, 1993). Studies like this reveal that deep down in our
most primitive nature, beauty is a form of communication that indicates something is
of good quality. It is transmitted subconsciously. And we like beauty because it makes

us feel good or euphoric. This is a key component of understanding beauty and why we covet it.

This internal wiring of the human brain sparks a positive emotional response to beauty. Recently I took my oldest daughter, Ari, to the Chicago Museum of Contemporary Art, and while we both were staring at an abstract floor display of a paper clip, she asked me, "Daddy, what makes this art beautiful?" That was a tough one, but after giving it some thought, I asked her, "How does it make you feel?" I told her, "For something to be beautiful to you it has to make you feel good, and if you have to think about whether or not it's beautiful, it probably isn't." She glanced at me for a second and then asked if we could go to the American Girl Store.

> Concepts of beauty aren't manufactured by Madison Avenue— infants as young as three months can recognize beautiful faces and stare at them longer than less beautiful ones.

The biggest impact of beauty takes place below the surface—if we're unsure about a feature and have to think about it, the purpose is lost. Just as we derive pleasure from monetary rewards and certain smells and sounds, neurological studies have shown that when we *visualize* something aesthetically pleasing, the reward centers in our brains are stimulated. In contrast, if we are asked to examine an object to determine if it is beautiful, the stimulation of the same reward centers is diminished. Our pleasure is reduced if we have to consciously evaluate the image (Winston, O'Doherty, Kilner, Perrett & Dolan, 2007).

In a study to prove this phenomenon, people were asked to look at photos of predetermined attractive men and women and judge their age and attractiveness level. During the judgment phase, researchers performed an MRI to measure each subject's brain activity. While judging the age of the attractive images, the reward centers in the subjects' brains were stimulated, but when they were asked to evaluate the images specifically for attractiveness, their major reward centers fired less strongly. So to reiterate this, because I believe it is an important distinction, when looking at the photos and judging age the evaluators were not focusing in on the attractiveness levels of the people in the photo yet their pleasure centers were stimulated, However when asked to judge the attractiveness levels of the photographed men and women the evaluators pleasure centers were underwhelmed. Wow, these findings were paradoxically unexpected, but suggest that beauty has the greatest impact when we don't think about it consciously. The pleasure comes when beauty is communicated and recognized in our deepest wiring.

> Beauty has the greatest impact when we don't have to think about it consciously.

This was the "aha!" moment for me! After realizing what this study meant to me and my profession I felt like I was given the secret decoder to understanding what is beautiful.

It boils down to how you perceive it and the way you feel when witnessing it. In other words, if you have to think about whether something is beautiful, it isn't.

And this goes beyond the perception of a pretty face, pleasure centers in our brain are teased and stimulated when we subconsciously perceive something as beautiful, whether it is a Monet painting, a sparkling daffodil, or the symmetric Taj Mahal. It is natural and human nature to want to please ourselves and this is precisely what beauty does for us.

The Impact of "Fake" Beauty

Last summer we took the kids to Paris for a family wedding. While there, I wanted them to see the most famous painting in the world, the *Mona Lisa* at the Louvre museum. I knew the girls would see many renditions of the legendary painting in their lifetime and I thought they would appreciate seeing the original. Against their wishes, I brought them to the museum and made them walk a long distance until they finally got to the large crowd of people gathered around the iconic painting. They were quite disappointed and unimpressed. It seemed much smaller than they thought and they weren't sure what was so special about it. My oldest daughter asked me what made it so great, so I read her the guide book's notes on the uniqueness of DaVinci's creation, but it clearly went over her head—and I think mine as well.

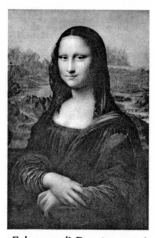

Fake or real? Does it matter?

The questions kept coming, such as: "Why is it different from the one we see at La Rosas, the Italian restaurant back home?"

"Well, this is the original, and that one is a copy," I said.

And that made me wonder. What if you didn't know—what if the Louvre switched out DaVinci's original for the copy back at La Rosas in Skokie? Would it matter? In fact, this premise was tested in a study that asked fourteen observers (untrained in art) to look at a Rembrandt painting. The investigators told them that the painting was either authentic or a copy. The catch was that sometimes they looked at an authentic and were told it was a copy, and other times they observed a copy and were told it was the real thing. Those who were told it was real showed stimulation in their brain reward centers, regardless of whether the painting was real or fake! All that mattered was that the observer *believed* it was real (Kemp & Parker, 2011).

I've seen the same thing play out in real life many times, including an example close to home. My dad has the interesting habit of transferring an inexpensive jug of wine into an impressive crystal decanter and serving it to guests as if it were a select Rothschild reserve from 1945. He doesn't lie about the name but simply tells them he is pouring them his favorite French wine. Granted, I don't think any of dad's friends are expert wine connoisseurs, but everybody is quick to comment on how great the wine tastes.

> Our brain reward centers sizzle when we think we're looking at a famous original work of art—whether it's a fake or not. All that matters is that we believe it's real.

I understand where my dad's frugal and practical mentality comes from. A native of Morocco, he grew up in Europe with eight siblings and was very street savvy by the time he emigrated to the United States at age twenty with little financial means. Over the years he came to enjoy

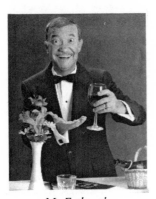

many of the finer things in life, including wine, and prefers the jug table-wine variety that he buys in bulk, because he says it tastes great and the price is right. Still, every time I'm at his house enjoying a formal dinner with guests I take him aside and gently challenge him on this practice.

He says, "What's the difference? They enjoy it nonetheless."

Growing up, I thought my dad's palate must be rather unsophisticated when it comes to wine, but now I wonder if actual "quality" is the best gauge of how much pleasure something brings us. How much does

My Father the wine enthusiast

it truly matter if it is real or authentic? And even if something is genuine, the real thing, but you tell people it's not, does it surprise you to hear they won't enjoy it as much.

Let's take water, for instance.

If I asked you what does water tastes like, what would you say? Most people have a hard time describing it. But Americans spend billions of dollars a year on bottled water because they think it tastes better. Now it may be a good idea to drink bottled water when you're traveling in certain foreign countries, because the local water may have different bacterial flora than you're accustomed to and it's a safer choice for your digestive system. But if we put your local tap water into a bottle, would you know the difference? Probably

> Beauty is as Beauty Seems: If I can help someone appear younger or more attractive in a subtle, authentic way, and unknowing observers are not privy to the method, they are rewarded with a pleasurable experience much the same as if that person were naturally youthful or beautiful.

not, because nearly half of the bottled water sold in the United States is tap water (*Food & Water Watch*)!

Anything can be made more impressive by the way we describe and laud it because our beliefs are as powerful as our instincts. This may be more relevant to modern art, where if there were no explanation or interpretation provided it may be hard for the untrained observer to decide if the paperclip on the ground is treasure or trash. Critics and other trusted authorities give us information that is strongly influential.

The same applies to beauty and plastic surgery. If I can help someone appear younger or more attractive in a subtle, authentic way, and unknowing observers are

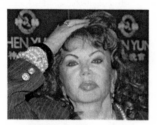

Jackie Stallone with what some may consider too much make up

not privy to the method, they are rewarded with a pleasurable experience much the same as if that person were naturally youthful or beautiful. But if an observer is tipped off that someone is unnaturally enhanced, he/she is no longer rewarded with the pleasure that beauty imparts. In fact, they often have a negative response to the altered appearance.

Consider how some women put on excessive makeup to highlight rosy cheeks, thick red lips or larger eyes, or wear clothing that is too tight in an attempt to highlight curves, or too much perfume to accentuate a sexy smell. While all of these are attempts to highlight femininity, what they actually communicate is the woman's attempt to overcompensate for a lack of natural beauty traits. Science proves it.

French researchers assessing perceptions of women with makeup professionally placed found that the women will be positively perceived, however, when placed in excess, make up can evoke negative responses (Richetin, Croizet & Huguet, 2004). Others also have shown that makeup, when applied inappropriately or excessively, can trigger negative impressions (Lewis & Bowler, 2009; Workman & Johnson, 1991). The message observers receive is that the person who applies too much makeup is not vital, healthy, or the possessor of good genes. It has the exact opposite effect of what the woman is trying to achieve! The same can be seen with excess plastic surgery.

> Inappropriate or excessive makeup is a turn-off, sending a message that the person is not vital, healthy, or the possessor of good genes.

Natural-looking beauty is best, and obvious enhancements are detrimental. We appreciate and gain pleasure from something that is beautiful when we believe it is the real thing. But what is the real thing?

Nature's Foundations of Beauty

As part of my quest to find the common traits of human beauty, I traveled to India to see the Taj Mahal, built in the seventeenth century by Emperor Shah Jahan as a memorial to his wife who died in childbirth. It was an unforgettable experience. The beauty of this architectural masterpiece from both a distance and up close is indescribable. It completely

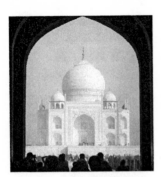

overwhelmed my senses and struck a pang in my soul as I stared at it with my eyes wide open. Unsurprised, my guide looked at me and said, "There are only two types of people in this world—those who have seen the Taj Mahal and those who have not."

The Taj Mahal's beauty is a result of many aspects of design that evoke pleasure, including one that plays an important role in human beauty: symmetry. The breathtaking balance of the Taj Mahal's proportions, minarets and mirrored reflection in the pool that lies in front of it echoes the symmetry we are programmed to find attractive in a human face.

The perfect symmetry of the Taj Mahal

Symmetry

While there is some debate among scientists regarding how much influence each tenet of beauty holds, it seems to boil down to four major traits. The first is symmetry.

Whether in art, nature or human beings, the more symmetric an object, the more favorably it is perceived. Why? From the lowliest insects to complex mammals, like humans, the brain likes symmetry because it can process it fluently and quickly. And the brain *likes* what is can process quickly (Reber, Schwarz & Winkielman, 2004). Beauty signals are sent to the amygdala, pre-frontal cortex and other

> The brain likes symmetry because it can process it fluently and quickly.

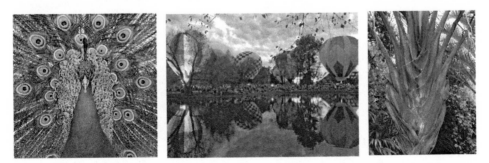

Symmetry throughout nature is attractive and in living creatures indicates health.

primitive parts of the brain, which light up when we evaluate something beautiful, whether it's the Taj Mahal or the perfect proportions of Grace Kelly's face.

Think of our brain's ability to process symmetry like a game that challenges you to spot the difference between two seemingly identical objects. Picking out the variations is tough because the brain is designed to quickly scan for balance. Similarly, the less symmetric an object is, the longer your brain takes to process it and the less pleasure it enjoys as a result.

Nowhere is the issue of symmetry more important than with the central portion of the face (Springer et al., 2007). We start the process of scanning an object from the center out, therefore a mole near the middle of the face is often considered unattractive but when located toward the outside of the face found attractive. It becomes a beauty mark when it occurs on the cheek or outside portion of the lip, but not when it is near the middle of the lip, chin, or forehead. For example, Marilyn Monroe's beauty mark on her left cheek is more beautifying than Cindy Crawford's signature mole near her upper lip.

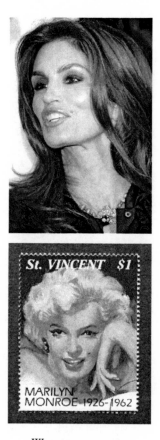

As we process symmetry in the face, we start in the middle and work our way out, and for both men and women the nose is the first stop in defining facial symmetry. We don't like signs of asymmetry near the middle part of the face and this is why a nose is so essential to the perception of our appearance. The nose as the leading feature on a face and one of the first features to be noticed by others, and a key element to defining facial symmetry.

A nose that is highly asymmetric projects an unhealthy impression and is more likely to capture an observer's subconscious attention. This detraction may prevent us from looking at the eyes, which is the most desirable place to look. In my practice, after nasal reshaping surgery, it is very common to hear from patients that they are suddenly receiving comments about their beautiful eyes and rarely hear a thing about their nose. If the nose procedure is done well, it should be

We process symmetry from the middle of the face and work our way out. Because we don't like signs of asymmetry near midline, we perceive a mole or beauty mark near the middle of the lip, chin, or forehead, as less beautiful than one that appears further from the middle, like Marilyn Monroe's.

> The key to expressing a beautiful feature is to make it unnoticeable and subconsciously communicated.

unnoticeable and blend into the rest of the face, allowing attention to naturally flow toward the eyes, where beauty is most commonly communicated. If a nose is surgically changed but looks obviously altered or overdone, it can have the opposite effect and suggest an unhealthy impression. *The key to expressing a beautiful feature is to make it unnoticeable and subconsciously communicated.*

Those who say they can always spot someone who has had a facelift frequently mention the obvious scars around the ears and the unnatural pull along the jaw line. However, rarely do people come to my clinic to fix these "branded" signs. And I am always surprised that they are barely, if at all, disturbed by these telltale marks of plastic surgery. The reason is that most people don't closely scrutinize their ears or the region on the sides of their face.

If I were to ask you if your ears look the same, would you know? Many people don't realize that their ears are highly asymmetric. When looking at someone else or even ourselves, we usually focus on the central part of the face. So, a person is often unconcerned and unfazed by an unsightly mole or scar by their ear.

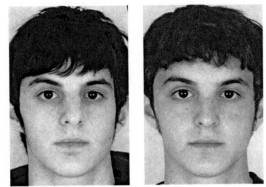

Blonde or not, the symmetric have more fun because there are many advantages to facial symmetry. In the animal kingdom, those with a higher

Many patients who undergo rhinoplasty (nasal reshaping surgery) say that they receive comments about their eyes. Making the nose more symmetrical naturally allows the eyes to become the focal point.

amount of symmetry are more likely to mate earlier and survive longer. In the plant world, the more symmetric a flower, the more likely it will be visited by bees and produce a greater amount of nectar. For male and female humans, the more facially symmetric, the more likely they are to have sex earlier. Symmetry is preferred throughout nature because it indicates that an individual is healthy, parasite-free, and less likely to harbor disease. Throughout nature, both in the animal and plant kingdoms, symmetry correlates with being healthy and is therefore seen as attractive. But why?

> Symmetry is preferred throughout nature because it indicates that an individual is healthy, parasite-free, and less likely to harbor disease.

All highly evolved organisms have a paired genetic DNA code that works much like a blueprint for our bodily organs, appendages, and characterizing physical traits. During fetal development, our genetic blueprints, except in rare situations, design the two sides of our body to be mirror images. Basically, we are all born with a genetic DNA blueprint that should code for complete symmetry.

In a perfect world, we would all be completely symmetric, but as we develop both in the womb and early out of the womb our bodies are bombarded with stressors from the environment such as disease, trauma, malnutrition, weather, and a thousand other little things that our developing bodies need to spend valuable internal resources fighting off. When we dedicate valuable energy to those challenges instead of using it to fulfill our genetic blueprint for perfect symmetry, that development is compromised, and one side of the face or body may not look exactly like the other.

Think of it like this. Imagine you're stranded in the remote Alaskan wilderness and winter is looming. You realize that soon it will be dark, cold, and sleeting. Are you more likely to build a shelter made of nearby branches and leaves that will keep you warm, but lacks any convenient amenities, or take the time and energy to build a plush log cabin? Sure, the beautiful log cabin sounds nice, but you probably wouldn't survive to finish it. You would more likely build the quick shelter, but if you had endless time and resources, were well rested, fed, and full of energy, you may decide to build that beautiful and showy log cabin. Similarly, the human organism has to use its energy to defend itself from the elements of viruses, parasites, and bacteria before it can worry about a perfect showy smile. And if any living organism does have a glamorous exterior, it would be the peacock with a fabulous symmetric tail which indicates it has an abundance of healthy internal resources and can afford to devote some of its extra energy to developing a pretty outside.

> The fact that nature wants symmetric-looking males to procreate more often than other men doesn't excuse a married man's philandering, but it goes a long way in explaining it.

In nature, it's survival first, beauty second.

That's why a lack of symmetry is a subconscious clue indicating diminished health. Theoretically, a very symmetric male possesses good, healthy genes—therefore, females are more interested in mating with them. Would you believe it if I told you a woman is more likely to orgasm when having sex with a symmetric man? Of eighty-six heterosexual couples who were asked details about their sex lives by a team of doctors at the University of New Mexico, the women who had intercourse with more symmetrical men achieved orgasms more often (Thornhill, Gangestad & Comer, 1995). During a female orgasm, powerful vaginal and uterine contractions force sperm up into the fallopian tubes where they are more likely to fertilize an egg. A woman subconsciously knows when she is with a male who is genetically fit and superior, and by having an orgasm, she gives preference to his sperm to fertilize her egg.

But the unsettling news is that a male who is more symmetric is also less likely to be faithful to his female partner. If you can think of this is in the raw terms of evolution, nature desires males with the most symmetric features and therefore motivates them to procreate more often than those who are asymmetric. This doesn't excuse a married man's philandering, but it goes a long way in explaining it.

Nature vs. Extremes: Those with extremes in height, weight, or perhaps even intelligence and artistic talent at either end of the spectrum are less likely to survive, because nature considers being out in front making waves and taking risks as dangerous.

Averageness

Who would you say is the most beautiful female superstar? Halle Berry? Natalie Portman? Salma Hayek? Angelina Jolie? Kim Kardashian? Do you think these gorgeous women would have been considered the most beautiful in the 1950s or '60s?

Being "average" is another element in nature's blueprint of beauty. In biology this is known as *koniophilia*, the love of the average. The more common something is, the more likely it is to survive. Nature doesn't often favor extremes because average, from a genetic and evolutionary perspective, is a lot safer. Those with extremes in height, weight or perhaps even intelligence and artistic talent at either end of the spectrum are less likely to survive, because nature considers being out in front making waves and taking risks as dangerous. And although those who lead us and change the world and our perspectives are either revered or vilified, they are often the risk takers whom nature tends to lop off more easily. Such bold difference makers as Michael Jackson, Marilyn Monroe, Elvis Presley, Martin Luther King, Pocahontas, Alexander the Great, JFK, Princess Diana and many more may move the needle but their genius also seems to make them susceptible to paying the ultimate price frequently before their contributions are realized. Those who lead into battle or those at the back of the line are the first ones to die.

Every time I travel to a distant land I come back a

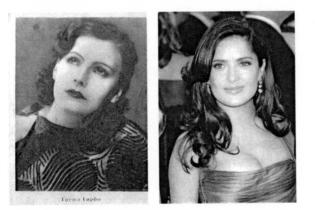

What we find to be a beautiful face has changed as our population become more ethnically diverse.

different person. It is with each stamp on my passport that I gather a new and different perspective further defining who and what I am. My sensitivities for the difference in cultures gains depth but the real return comes from my learned appreciation for the similarities within humankind. What I didn't realize is that I was also subconsciously resetting the physicality I find attractive. Nature selects for those who remain in the middle of the pack. Beauty, similarly, is most desirable when it reflects the average appearance of a population. The average looks most familiar and feels most comfortable to us.

If I were to drop you off in the middle of the Papa New Guinea forest, into an isolated tribe of natives where all the women have deeply dark skin, short hair, wear very little clothing, and have had minimal interaction with the "modern world," do you think you would be able to detect who is the most beautiful woman in the tribe? Or would you find that they all look the same? How about if I dropped you off in a remote region of northern Tibet near China—could you easily detect the most attractive female in the local culture? The answer is no, at first, but yes, later.

The brain processes the familiar more fluently than the foreign. It also finds the familiar more pleasing and beautiful. This is why many find their close friends and associates becoming increasingly attractive to them over time. It is the reason the person setting you up on a blind date with her best friend tells you with all honesty how attractive she is, when in reality she is rather uneasy on the eyes. It is also the reason that, when first encountering a foreign race, most people focus on the differences, such as skin color or eye shape, and find it difficult to find this new group of people attractive or to identify who is attractive within this population. "They all look the same." However, after the brain becomes familiar with these individuals, their skin color and facial architecture become part of the brain's reference section and we soon recognize the subtleties that make certain individuals attractive within their own population. Our brain then scans all the references in our system and morphs them together to find the mean or average appearance, and this appearance is what we find most attractive. But what is even more interesting is that when you return home from your extended stay in Papa New Guinea or Tibet, you will likely find a different type of person more attractive. Your overall perception of beauty has been tweaked by becoming familiar with the features common to the foreign culture.

> We're programmed to perceive the "average" look of a population as beautiful, because averageness means that the person possesses multiple unique gene combinations—making him or her more fit for survival. And in the U.S., "average" has shifted away from the mostly Caucasian look that Twiggy personified in the 1960s.

Attractive faces have been found to be the most average faces of a population (Langlois & Roggman, 1990). It is genetically intuitive that the average appearance of the population would be most desirable or found most beautiful, because this suggests that the individual has the most diverse gene combination. In other words, the most average-looking people have the benefit of multiple unique gene combinations, which gives them the ability to adapt or survive in any environment. Following this theory, it is not surprising that children born of two parents from very different genetic backgrounds and races are often very attractive. Can anyone say Halle Berry? The best of their genes come together to create an offspring that is better equipped to survive and thrive. It's the same reason children of incest or closed communities with a high percentage of inbreeding tend to have more disease and be unattractive. Nature wants us to mate with someone who has very different genes from our own.

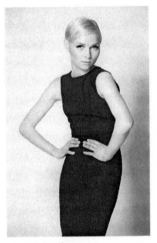

Therefore, in a multicultural population, the average of society is the most beautiful; while in a homogenous population the ideals of beauty possess character traits that are consistent with the entire population. For example, in the 1960s, the British model Twiggy represented ideal female beauty in America.

She possessed an infantile face with large round eyes, high eyebrows, a small up-turned nose, thin lips, and narrow jaw. At the time, the U.S. population was eighty-five percent Caucasian with relatively little Asian, Latin, or African influence. Today, American society is far

Models often try to recreate Twiggy's 1960s look.

more multicultural and the average has become a blend of character traits from these cultures. What is considered beautiful today is a face with features that reflect these ethnic influences such as a heavier brow, larger nose, and thicker lips. Rather than the very Anglo beauty of the 1960s, today's beauties are the likes of Angelina Jolie, Salma Hayek, and Jennifer Lopez.

When I was in medical school, we were still studying the ideal canons of facial perfection described by sixteenth-century master Leonardo da Vinci.

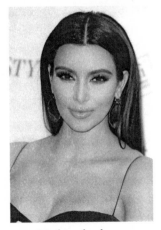

His recorded standards of beauty and ideal facial proportions are very Caucasian and Eurocentric, however, and not representative of our modern multicultural world. But there is evidence that a beautiful

Modern day beauty

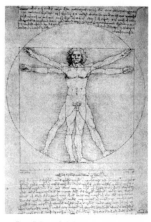

Da Vinci's Vitruvian man

face can be mathematically determined for each person regardless of ethnicity based on the distance between the inner corners of each eye and the Phi formula (1.618). (Swift and Remington 2011)Phi is known as the divine formula and is named after the Greek sculptor Phidias who described its use. However, the divine formula dates back to Ancient Egyptian culture. And from nature to architecture to art and more this divine formula seems to be at the root of all that is defined as visually pleasing. Like others in my field, I too have developed a mathematical model that applies this formula to determine the ideal facial proportions for an individual. I can then superimpose a customized ideal facial image on to a photograph for each person and demonstrate what is necessary to achieve the perfect phi face. On occasion in the clinic or operating, I may refer to this model to confirm my treatment plan. And my phi model may prove particularly helpful for the person at home wanting to know where the most flattering position is for their hairline, cheek highlights or eyebrows. Additionally, I provide my model to make -up artists, medical students and physicians wanting to learn or better their outcomes in cosmetic treatments and surgery. However, is it my belief that an attractive face cannot be one dimensional and easily manufactured with the help of a tape measure. There is so much more depth to what makes a person feel beautiful and unfortunately, our cosmetic medical journals

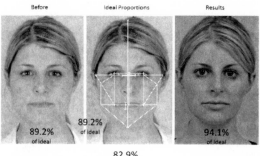

Dr. Dayan's Phi mathematical formula for beauty. Based only on the distance between the eyes the ideal location for the important features of the face (cheek highlights, nose, mouth and chin) can be determined for each person regardless of ethnicity. A face then can be compared to its ideal proportions for that individual and the physician or makeup artist can then be directed to where on the face certain features should be accentuated. For example a face may be 85% of the idealized face for that individual person but by slightly widening the eyes or filling the cheeks or narrowing the jawline the face may reach 95% of what the ideal face would be for that person. In the photo above the final result soon after treatment with non-surgical methods (neuromodulators (Botox), fillers (Restylane) and laser is achieved.

and textbooks in my opinion overemphasize the importance of evaluating the face using formulas and measurements. Yes, today's surgeons should know the Phi mathematical formulas of beauty because it is proving a good guide to making a face appear physically pleasing but more importantly to recognize and appreciate the difficult to define but ever present human element that resides at the core of beauty.

Youthfulness

At what age do you think a woman is found most beautiful, based on physical appearance alone? While in reality there is no such evaluation, because we view people as a composite of multiple characterizing traits, we can calculate the ideal facial age for beauty in computer simulation studies.

Nature favors the young because they represent the most promising and potential-filled period for any species, especially for females, so we are programmed to perceive youthfulness as beautiful. The more infantile a female's features, the more beautiful she is perceived. This was confirmed in a study in which computer composite photos of females from eighteen to thirty years in age were evaluated by men and women (Johnston, Solomon, Gibson & Pallares-Bejarano, 2003). Precise sites were marked on the photographed faces to determine the exact position and size of the lips, nose, chin, eyes, and other features. Afterward, the photos that the judges found most attractive were associated with large lips, a small chin, high hair, and large eyes—features strongly associated with younger women. The average age of the most beautiful faces was calculated to be 24.9 years. This correlated with the age males most desire in a female when considering a potential long-term relationship. A large study of thirty-seven cultures, which found men from all cultures desire women around the age of 24.8 years (Buss, Shackelford & LeBlanc, 2000).

> Nature Favors the Young: The more infantile a female's features—small chin, large lips, large eyes— the more beautiful she is perceived to be.

Cultures around the world share the perception that the youthful characteristics of high cheekbones, large eyes, a small chin, even-toned skin and plump lips are beautiful. A youthful and beautiful face draws attention to the eyes and assumes an inverted triangle with its greatest width at the cheeks and driving to a narrow point at the chin. As females age, the cheeks descend and form deep hollows around the eyes and the cheek fat pad falls over the jaw line, creating jowls. The chin becomes more square-like and the face begins to take on masculine characteristics. The human mind interprets these traits as aging, infertile, and of diminished attractiveness.

When evaluating a person at an initial encounter, where is the first place on their face you look? If you said the eyes, you are correct. Two lovers sit in a bar staring into each others eyes. What are they looking for? What signals are passing between them?

Youthful face Vs. Mature face

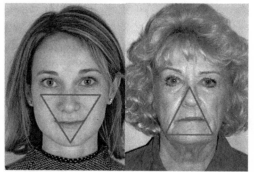

As females age the jaw becomes more square and the triangle of youth reverses.

As a source of subconscious messaging, beauty is incredibly persuasive and effective. And for the youthful face, beauty begins with the eyes. Men are attracted to big eyes in females, especially if the pupils are large, and this attraction is rooted in a female's normal physiological responses. When a woman is sexually stimulated or attracted in her fertile ovulatory phase, her pupils dilate. In a study done in Norway at the University of Tromsø, women were asked to look at photos of their boyfriends and famous male sex symbols. The women responded with a maximum pupil dilation of eight percent (Laeng & Falkenberg, 2007).

Those two lovers in a bar engaged in a deep conversation may not be aware that her pupils are dilating. However, his primitive brain centers pick up this subconscious signal and send a message to his conscious brain to become further engaged. If the female is on oral contraceptives, however, this phenomenon doesn't occur. Birth control pills mimic pregnancy, and theoretically a pregnant female would not be a good candidate for passing along one's genes, so there is no need to send a sexually advanced message to a male. A man would be better served directing his attention elsewhere where his energy and resources would be more likely to result in finding a mate who is fertile and ready to procreate. This is one of the reasons many men prefer blue eyes—dilating pupils are easier to see. A man can more quickly assess the pupillary changes and gauge the interest of a woman with blue eyes than a woman with dark eyes.

> A man can more easily see that a woman's pupils are dilating if the woman has blue eyes. In her ovulatory phase, a woman's pupils will dilate when she is sexually stimulated or attracted.

One of my patients who came in for nasal reshaping had a nose out of proportion to the rest of her features, but wow, did she have incredibly beautiful eyes.

I asked my medical students if they could tell me what was unique about her, and they didn't seem to know, other than that her nose was big. They all concluded she was attractive, but they didn't really know why. I explained that they were hard-wired to be attracted to her blue eyes and unusually large pupils. After the rhinoplasty, this patient mentioned, acquaintances couldn't tell what was different, but just kept commenting on her pretty eyes. I wasn't at all surprised when she told me about her new job as a sales manager for a luxury retailer.

Because the eyes play such an important role in attraction, makeup, cosmetic treatments and surgery devoted to highlighting the eyes are very popular throughout the world. And eye enhancement is nothing new: in the Middle Ages, belladonna (from the Italian meaning "beautiful woman") was a popular drug among women because it dilated the pupils. Knowing that men like large pupils, savvy medieval damsels placed drops of belladonna in their eyes when headed out on the town in a subtle attempt to attract a mate. The only problem was, they could barely see in bright light!

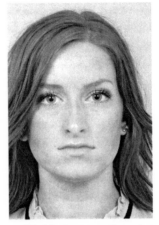

We like large pupils and light-colored eyes.

Many women intuitively know the benefits of enhancing the eyes, and this is one of the first areas of the face where women learn to use makeup. Almost seventy percent of women in the U.S. use mascara. Although eyes are the feature that shows the earliest signs of aging, they can easily be gently tweaked with a few minor procedures. This is likely why Botox, with its eye-enhancing effects, is the number-one cosmetic medical procedure in the world, and blepharoplasty (eyelid repair or reconstruction) one of the most common surgical procedures in the United States.

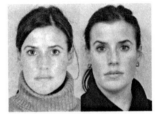

Botox can be used to make the eyes appear more open and inviting.

Advertisers and graphic artists are also keenly aware that dilated pupils are the key to making a female more attractive, and may alter the images in their ads accordingly. Take a close look inside some of the magazines on your desk and you will see how many images include this technique. Disney® and Mattel® are also privy to the attractive powers of large pupils, as seen in their female cartoon characters and Barbie dolls.

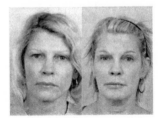

Blepharoplasty (eyelid lifts) improves the appearance of the eyes.

If a man wants to know if a female is subconsciously sending a signal that she is interested, all he has to do is peer into her eyes and discover if her pupils are dilated. The eyes tell all, and facial aesthetic strategies are directed toward highlighting the eyes. One way for a woman to let a man know that she's interested without being obvious is to keep her eyes open and inviting. This is a conscious way of mimicking dilated pupils. But she has to be careful

> One way for a woman to let a man know that she's interested without being obvious is to keep her eyes open and inviting.

not to overdo it—a surprised look puts the man on the defensive instead of drawing him in.

Interestingly, men and women differ when it comes to increasing the attractive appearance of the eyes. The more contrast between the color around the eyes and the surrounding skin, the more attractive a woman's eyes appear, which explains the development of eyeliner and makeup shades to highlight femininity. But for a man it's the opposite. If he has dark, deep-set eyes, a woman perceives this as a sign of aggression. In fact, certain characteristics such as contrast around the eyes or position of the brow may make one gender appear more attractive and the other less so.

These curious differences in characterizing features are defined as being sexually dimorphic, meaning that the trait is divergently opposite for each gender. Therefore, the darker the eyes and lighter the skin, the more feminine an appearance becomes. However, the more similar in color the eyes are to the skin, the more masculine one appears. And sexually dimorphic traits when expressed in the appropriate gender have developed to become recognized signs of beauty. From a biological perspective, someone who strongly exhibits the sexually dimorphic trait signals that he or she carries good genes. To apply this to treatment for women, my practice includes tools for highlighting and accentuating the appearance of the

> In every race and culture, females are noted to be more light-skinned than males. Lighter skin allows a woman to produce more Vitamin D, which is essential for strong bones and healthy pregnancies.

eyes as compared to the surrounding skin. Increasing the contrast between the eyes and surrounding skin will make the eyes "pop," resulting in a more attractive and engaging female appearance.

Flawless Skin

I recently gave a lecture to over 300 senior high school students from the Chicago Public schools. I was talking about the importance of avoiding too much sun and how it cannot only lead to skin cancer, but also premature aging of the skin. So, to further illustrate the damaging effects of excess sun exposure, I showed the students two bananas, one that was riddled with darkly spotted and dull skin and another that was bright yellow. I asked the students which of the bananas was older, and they immediately shouted out something about the darker one. I then showed them a close-up photo of the facial skin of someone who had been an abuser of sun tanning booths for many years and had a very mottled appearance. Next to that photo I showed a picture of someone with well-cared-for skin. I then asked them which person was more youthful, and they all pointed to the latter photo.

> We have evolved to perceive a man's darker skin and a woman's lighter skin as beautiful.

Just like the banana, youthful skin has an even tone and color. These external features are associated with internal fitness and female hormone estrogen levels (Thornton, 2002). When one is healthy and young, the skin color is translucent and clear. Blood pumped to the skin reflects light, resulting in a healthy pinkish hue. During the aging process, wrinkles form, skin loses it tone, and facial fat atrophies or disappears.

Skin color is a sexually dimorphic trait; females in all cultures are noted to be a few shades lighter than the males of their culture. The female's lighter skin of youth has an evolutionary purpose as it allows in more sunlight, which helps the body manufacture vitamin D, an essential ingredient for strong bones and important for pregnancy. However, once a woman has a child and starts the aging process, her skin begins to darken.

Males also have an evolutionarily adaptive reason for their darker skin. Men who were often out on the hunt were exposed to more daytime sun and required darker skin to protect them from the sun's damaging rays. Therefore, we have evolved to perceive a man's darker skin and a woman's lighter skin as beautiful. The effects of pregnancy and years of sun exposure cause the aging facial skin to show dark spots, rough patches, and tiny blood vessels known as spider veins or telangiectasias, all of which cause the skin to lose its sheen. These are all signs of the aging process and/or disease.

There is strong evidence that the skin's appearance is a clue into our internal fitness.

Signs of disease, such as yellow skin, can occur with jaundice or liver disease, while anemia is associated with an overly pale appearance. In addition, skin changes occur with vitamin and hormonal deficiency, thyroid disease, and numerous other ailments. The unknowing eye of the observer picks this up as a subconscious clue that indicates aging or disease. From an evolutionary perspective, someone seeking a potentially good mate would question whether this is a suitable person to pursue.

Dark spots appearing on the skin as we age are a natural process, just like the brown spots that show up on fruit and vegetables when they become overripe. Many people who come to my office know that they want

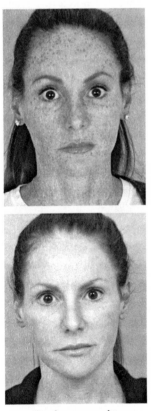

Dark spots on skin indicate aging and can be reversed with lasers.

Before there were blood tests, our primitive ancestors looked for external clues in someone's facial appearance to determine that person's health. We're still deeply wired to do the same.

to look younger, but they can't pin down exactly what needs to be changed. When we look at an older person, three specific features are quickly equated with aging: an elongated upper lip, wrinkled and mottled skin, and gray hair. In a study done comparing the age appearances between twins, it was found that these three signs had the greatest impact on subconsciously signaling to others the aging process (Gunn et al. 2009). So, if you believe you are looking older but aren't quite sure why, you may want to take a look at these three areas. In a follow-up twin study, the twin that looked older had a higher mortality rate. In other words, looking older correlated with dying earlier (Christensen et al., 2004).

Our facial appearance, then, is a strong indicator of our internal health. This was further confirmed in a study in 2000 that evaluated over 400 civil servants in London. Observers noted that grey hair made women look older, which was no surprise (Bulpitt, Markowe & Shipley, 2001), but blood tests revealed that the gray-haired women showed higher levels of inflammation. Signs of internal disease show up in our skin and hair, causing us to appear unhealthy, older, and therefore less attractive.

The research findings on disease and aging are rather consistent. Before there were blood tests and X-rays to determine our internal health, our primitive ancestors looked for external clues in facial appearance to determine a person's health. And one day in the not-so-distant future, can you imagine walking up to a kiosk, having your face scanned by a computer and based on your facial appearance accurately determine the status of your health? Physical appearance and the impression we project are clearly linked to our age and internal health.

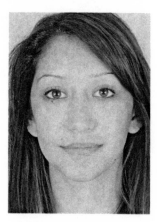

A youthful face appears to represent health and fertility

Youthful Lips

Large lips send a strong fertility symbol, which is why they are so often equated with a beautiful face. The male's subconscious mind associates large lips with fertility because they correspond with the appearance of the genitals, which swell during ovulation. A fertile female has full, red lips framed by a distinctive white border. The lips of youth engorge ever so slightly during the height of female fertility and reach their greatest size around age 14 to an average of 19.4 mm (Farkas & Cheung, 1981). In a study in which males identified the size of lips they found most attractive, they chose the female photos with lips at 19.4 mm (Johnston et al., 2003). When a woman puts on lipstick or seductively enhances her lips, she may not realize that she's sending a subconscious message to the primitive male mind that she is fertile and ovulating.

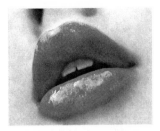

Fertile full lips are attractive and signal fertility.

The Curvy Ratio

If a naked woman stands in front of a man, what part of her body do you thing he looks at first?

I have a first cousin who is very good looking and eligible. He seeks out women like a Beagle does food. He usually dates models and movie stars, but recently he asked me to fix him up with a girl who at first glance most women wouldn't consider attractive. In fact, my female staff members were shocked to hear that he had interest in her. She was shorter than average at just under five feet, and a bit heavy, but what they overlooked were the features that my cousin noticed first—her voluptuous curves. She has large, shapely breasts; a full behind and big lips; and instead of being a concern, her little belly pouch only added to her allure. This woman oozes fertility and men instantly recognize it. Men are driven to seek shapeliness and it is the midriff area that best defines a woman's curves.

> Men go crazy for hourglass figures because pregnancy-ready hips that carry a healthy layer of fat tell the primitive male mind that there are enough reserves to nurture an offspring.

Where do men look first?

The relationship between waist and hip size is what really piques a man's interest. Men are highly attracted and attuned to this area of the female body because it reveals much to a male's subconscious mind. The midriff of a potential mate can be accurately assessed from any direction and from long distances, no matter which direction the female is positioned, forward, back, or diagonally. In contrast, other healthy features of good genes such as a beautiful face or breasts can only be seen when viewing the person from the front. Additionally, whether shaded by clouds or silhouetted by the sun, a male can identify and detect within 200 milliseconds the curves of a female body and quickly determine her ability to procreate. In an eye-tracking study done in New Zealand in which males viewed rapidly shown photos of naked females on a computer screen, the

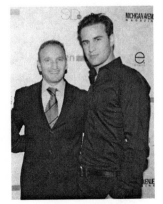

My very eligible cousin and me

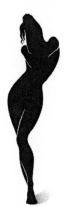

Where do men look first?

area they looked at first was not the eyes or genitalia, but the midriff section, from just below the breasts to the hips. (Dixson, Grimshaw, Linklater & Dixson, 2011).

What is it that the single-minded males are so interested in? The male mind is wired to seek out a waist-to-hip ratio between 0.65 and 0.75—in other words, a waist that is 65 to 75 percent the size of the hips. A female waist-to-hip ratio of 0.70 represents the curvilinear hourglass relationship that men find so sexy and attractive. The male subconscious mind likes this curvy ratio because—you guessed it— it is a powerful signal of fertility.

As a female enters puberty and becomes sexually mature, her surge of female hormones causes her hips to gain fat and width. Pregnancy-ready hips that carry a healthy layer of fat tell the primitive male mind that there are enough reserves to nurture an offspring (Zaadstra et al., 1993). Women with the ideal waist-to-hip ratio have body fat distribution consistent with greater health and reproductive potential (Singh, 1993), and higher estrogen and progesterone levels—important hormones for conception—also correlate to larger breasts and a narrow waist (Jasienska, Ziomkiewicz, Ellison, Lipson & Thune, 2004). Another study found that artificially inseminated females with optimal waist-to-hip ratios become pregnant more often and more quickly (Grammer, Fink, Moller & Thornhill, 2003).

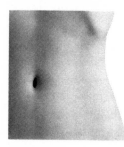

Men look at waist-to-hip ratio first to assess fertility.

The waist-to-hip ratio is a reliable signal about female reproductive status, reproductive capability, overall health, and perhaps the risks for major disease. Women with a very high waist-to-hip ratio (their waist is similar to or bigger than the width of their hips) have more difficulty in becoming pregnant (Kaye, Folsom, Prineas, Potter & Gapstur, 1990) and are more likely to have diseases, which makes them a poor risk for a male on the lookout for a mate to bear his children.

A smaller waistline helps draw attention to the areas where men look next, the buttocks and breasts, which are also sources of fat storage associated with fertility. Men don't really care about how much a woman weighs or how much fat she possesses, just as long as it is situated in the right proportions. In some cases, more tailored, fitted clothing or better posture is enough to create the illusion of the right proportions. Contrary to the super-thin look of runway models, a woman does not have to be a size two to be attractive. In some cultures, especially the less developed ones, as long as she possesses an ideal waist to hip ratio, a heavier female is actually more desired.

Money, Hunger, and Desire

A man's standard of beauty can be fickle, depending on whether he's on his way in or out of a restaurant.

That's right—men will change their desire for female heaviness based on their appetite. And their bank account.

In an interesting study done at New York University and Stanford, over 1,000 undergraduate men and women were surveyed about how much money they had in their pockets and bank accounts, and then asked questions about their ideal mate and body weight. The researchers learned that the less financially well-off men preferred the heavier females. An even more interesting finding was that hungry undergraduate men polled on their way to the dining hall also preferred a heavier female, when compared to the preferences of satiated males leaving the room (Nelson & Norton, 2005).

Men, therefore, base what they find attractive on their minute-to-minute feelings of hunger and their financial status. This individual preference can be extrapolated to a macro level to explain why in lower socioeconomic cultures and poorer countries, heavier females are found attractive. It is precisely in these resource-depleted environments that a well-rounded female would be a strong indicator to a prowling male that she possesses enough fat to get pregnant and support a baby. It is understandable then why obesity is more prevalent in communities where men seem to be more accepting of overweight women as attractive and sexy (Harris, Walters & Waschull, 1991).

> From caveman drawings to the Renaissance, the ideal waist-to-hip ratio has always been admired and glorified.

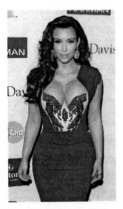

Kim Kardashian with an ideal waist-to-hip ratio

With the midriff and waist-to-hip ratio so critical to the male perspective of beauty and attractiveness, it's not surprising that the number-one cosmetic plastic surgery procedure in the U.S. is liposuction, which is an attempt to redistribute fat in order to achieve more ideal proportions. It's also why curvaceous stars like as Kim Kardashian and Jennifer Lopez continue to be sex symbols for men.

The ideal waist-to-hip ratio hasn't really changed in thousands of years. Even the classic painters, from the early Greeks to the Renaissance masters, appreciated the importance of the curvy ratio. A quick glance at the Venus de Milo reveals the ideal waist-to-hip ratio of 0.7. Although she appears quite buxom, from caveman drawings to the Renaissance, the ideal waist-to-hip ratio has always been admired and glorified. As another modern example, the waist-to-hip ratio for *Playboy* centerfolds and Miss America contestants has changed very little over a forty-year period. While the models in these magazines and contests have become slimmer, their hourglass shapes remained virtually the same, varying by only two percent (Singh, 1993)

The Female Obsession with Thinness

One recent winter I walked into the Hearst Building in New York City to be interviewed for a magazine article. I heard a rumbling in the lobby and then saw a strange gaggle of beings walking in a pack. At first I was overwhelmed by their shine, glitter, and bounce as they swayed toward the elevators, but I couldn't help noticing how strange this group appeared. They were very tall and thin with long necks and big heads that didn't fit their body size. They looked like

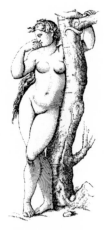

Even the masters recognized the importance of an attractive waist-to-hip relationship.

something out of a sci-fi movie, a gang of aliens right out of *ET the Extra-Terrestrial*. But then I realized that these women were runway models, the crème de la crème of female beauty, according to some standards. However, to a man's primitive mind, that couldn't be further from the truth.

The fascination with thinness may be a more female-derived concept, as it appears that women find this more attractive than men. Most men are attracted to a female with a feminine shape that is designed to produce offspring, and they actually find overweight and underweight women to be equally unattractive (Singh, 1993). This makes sense because obese women are associated with disease, while underweight women are more likely to become infertile. Males desire the curvy, fertile female, which is why male magazines such as *Maxim* and *Playboy* show very curvy women on their

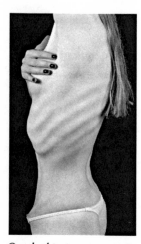

Overly thin is not attractive to the male's eyes.

The fascination with thinness may be a more female-driven concept, as it appears that women find this more attractive than men.

covers. Women, however, prefer to look at very slim shapes as reflected on the covers of magazines appealing to women's taste such as *Vogue*, *Cosmopolitan*, *Glamour*, and *Mademoiselle*, which over the years have shown increasingly thinner women with more revealing clothing (Sypeck, Gray & Ahrens, 2004).

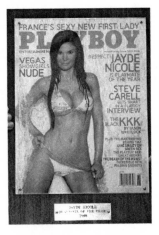

Magazines for each gender are specific to innate desires.

Are Vaginas Pretty?

I share my office space two days a week, with Dr. Otto Placik, who also happens to be my first cousin; his mom and my dad are siblings. Otto is a fantastic plastic surgeon who treats all parts of the body but in the last five years his practice has developed a special niche in female plastic surgery and vaginal rejuvenation in particular. He consults with women each week who are interested in labiaplasty, a procedure to reduce the size of the labia. The labia are the folds of tissue and skin that surround the opening to the vagina. As women enter puberty, their labia develop into different sizes and some expansion is normal and protective. But on occasion, the skin folds can be abnormally enlarged, leading to irritation and bleeding during walking or exercising. They may also become a noticeable aspect of a very private part of their body, even through clothing. In such cases, there may be a medical necessity to reducing their size. However, with today's newer bikini grooming trends, the labia are becoming more exposed and visible, and many women are seeking out labia reduction surgery for cosmetic reasons. But who are they doing it for?

We've learned that genitalia are not one of the first places a man looks when evaluating a female. There is no such thing as an ugly or pretty vagina. If anything, labia that are too small would be unattractive to the male eye because it would be more associated with a child than a fertile female. In the eye-tracking study mentioned above, in which men were confronted with photos of naked women, they did not look at the genitalia first, but instead at the midriff and breasts. The men's eye movements revealed that eighty percent of their first visual fixations were on the breast and midriff areas, the precise locations that define fertility (Dixson et al., 2011). As far as nature is concerned, the beauty that counts from a man's subconscious, mating-drive perspective isn't located in the bikini area. By the time he reaches the point of intimacy with a woman, it's unlikely a male is going to turn away—regardless of the appearance of the vagina.

> In one study, eighty percent of the men's visual fixations were on the breast and midriff areas, the precise locations that define fertility.

The foundations of beauty that count as universal attractors—symmetry, youth, averageness, and proportion—can each be enhanced to improve one's first impression. Rarely does someone possess all of them in their most ideal form. That kind of perfection is left to the Disney animators and Barbie doll designers. They may be perfect from a purely technical viewpoint, but a genuine portrait of human beauty? Not really. We're programmed to seek out health and vitality in a partner, not perfection.

CHAPTER 4

ARNOLD, MARIA AND THE HOUSEKEEPER

Viagra Triangle is a subset of the 'Rush Street' nightlife district on Chicago's Near North Side. So named for the abundance of mostly-affluent older men who frequent the local bars, and the 'triangle' where State and Rush Streets come together. The gentle ecosystem of the Viagra Triangle could not exist without a fully stocked pond of anxious and artificially infertile females. Seven years prior she may have been called a 'Trixie' in and around Lincoln Park, but with an East Bank membership, a Platinum card of her own, and several upgrades to the base Lexus, she is looking for more. —*Urban Dictionary*

I f he looks ultra-manly, he mostly likely has the robust genes to back it up.

But those dominant masculine traits and the primal urges that go with them make it tough going for alpha males in a world that admires manliness *and* monogamy.

In May of 2011, the *Los Angeles Times* broke the story that former Mr. Universe, Hollywood box office sensation and two-term California governor Arnold Schwarzenegger, admitted to having an affair and bearing a love child with his live-in house staffer. When his wife of twenty-five years, the elegant Maria Shriver, learned the news, including the fact that Arnold had been supporting his illegitimate son for ten years, she separated from

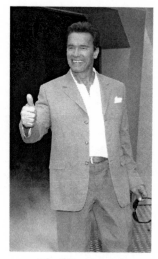

The "Governator"

him. Just as shocking as Arnold's at-home infidelity was his ability to keep the story under wraps for more than a decade, which is an eternity in politics. His mistress, who by Hollywood standards was neither beautiful nor physically fit, was also married at the time. Even more difficult to believe was that their love child was born five days after Maria gave birth to her and Arnold's fourth child. Maria, a member of the famed Kennedy clan, grew up hearing stories of infidelity involving her notorious uncle and former president John F. Kennedy, Jr., but to learn that her husband (who had been linked to many women during his time) had made her and another woman pregnant the same week was too much. She and Arnold eventually divorced.

Arnold is just the latest kingly politician to succumb to his drives—look no further than our forty-second President, William Jefferson Clinton, who found creative new ways to use a cigar along with stamping his brand forever into a famous blue dress. Others, such as U.S. Senator John Edwards, South Carolina Governor Mark Sanford, and Italian Prime Minister Silvio Berlusconi are perhaps the best-known politicians to have rocked the world with their affairs in recent times.

What drives such men to cheat when there's so much at stake if their affairs are discovered? Why do women become so enamored with men they perceive as powerful? Is this behavior wrong, or destined? Is it possible that just as humans are driven to crave sweets and must discipline themselves to not over indulge, powerful men are evolutionarily driven to desire multiple mates, and women feel biologically compelled to seek out powerful men?

> Is it possible that powerful men are evolutionarily driven to desire multiple mates, and women feel biologically compelled to seek out powerful men?

Perhaps we shouldn't be surprised at all over the exploits of men like Arnold and Bill. As Hugh Hefner so eloquently put it when Tiger Woods admitted to having affairs with several women simultaneously:

> "I think the only surprise in it, quite frankly, is that anybody would be surprised. If you're a good-looking guy and young and healthy, the notion that there would be something else going on, well, marriage is just a convenience. It's very nice for raising kids, but the notion that monogamy lasts forever is a wish!"

Anyone who has children would have trouble denying that boys and girls are very different. My three girls, ages thirteen, eleven and nine, play, don't socialize and interact with each other like boys their age do. The girls and their friends love to discuss who is being nice to whom and who is not, and to express feelings of rejection and denigration. They are very verbal, descriptive and sensitive. In contrast, boys are more physical, less talkative, and do not appear to be as deeply affected by their friends' actions.

> Based on the benefits of close cooperation with other women during childbearing years, women evolved to be empathetic and sociable.

Many of these distinct differences between young girls and boys are rooted in adaptive traits that developed over millions of years of evolution. They have been finely honed to allow our species to survive and thrive. In the harsh environment of primitive life, in which our species has spent ninety-nine percent of its evolution, the successful male is defined by his ability to provide resources for his mate and offspring until they reach an age of self-sufficiency. There were no grocery stores or contraception on the Pleistocene savannah. Therefore, an adult female would likely be pregnant, breastfeeding, or otherwise taking care of her offspring most of the time. She would not significantly contribute to garnering food or creating shelter. Moreover, while her male mate was away hunting for food, a pregnant female would greatly benefit from the assistance of other women in the community. She needed to be empathic and sociable.

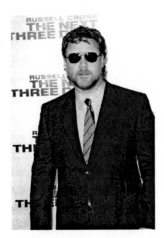

The Alpha Male

Gladiator, the Oscar-winning movie of 2000, stars the handsome and strapping Russell Crowe as Maximus, a wronged Roman warrior whose strength and courage intimidated those in power. Brutally robbed of his family and his freedom, he followed his new destiny and became the greatest gladiator in Rome. Many films share this focus on the lone hero battling the odds—think of Robert Redford in *The Natural*, Tom Cruise as Ethan Hunt, Daniel Craig as James Bond, Sylvester Stallone as Rambo, and Brad Pitt as Billy Beane in *Moneyball*.

All these characters are a similar type: the tormented male soul with enormous leadership skills, drive, and physical prowess who has loved, lost, and is forced to swim upstream. His children were taken from him or he

As Maximus in the movie Gladiator, Russell Crowe embodies the timeless traits of the alpha male: physical prowess and strength, courage, leadership, a go-it-alone attitude and intelligence.

is too busy saving the world to bond with the children he loves. The alpha male is a solitary creature who best handles and disposes of danger alone. But where does this attractive character come from, and why are we so drawn to him?

Do Superman and Barbie dolls appeal to boys and girls because they trigger a natural wish to be like them? Just like fashion magazines airbrush our female figures to appear flawless; our media constructs a male that can withstand any harsh environment. Both caricatures are appealing because they align with a very primitive human concept that has been shared throughout humanity across the ages.

> Males that develop and take on roles of leadership and physical prowess often possess physical clues into their ability to supply ample resources, such as a strong torso, dominant facial features, and powerful legs.

The alpha male is a hunter on a mission to bring home resources, which over hundreds of thousands of pre-civilized years most commonly meant food. A male who is very skilled at this task would likely possess physical adaptations that would make him highly efficient at bringing home the meat. He would probably be aerobically fit to chase down his prey, possess a sharp intellect to know how to track an animal, and be strong enough to fend off an attacking beast or jealous competitor bent on taking away what he has earned.

If I asked you to describe the physical appearance of an alpha male, what image pops into your mind's eye? Is he young or old, balding or sporting a full head of hair, tall or short? Most likely, your vision is similar to everyone else's. We all have a strong and consistent idea of what the alpha male looks like, because his qualities have been ingrained in us over hundreds of thousands of years. Males that develop and take on roles of leadership and physical prowess often possess physical clues into their ability to supply ample resources such as a strong torso, dominant facial features, and powerful legs. We all know a Superman when we see one. Our male heroes may get knocked down, but they pick themselves up and race onward in their mission to save the world. The practical advantages of those traits make sense, but why and where does the drive of so many men to go it alone come from?

Historically it has been the male's responsibility to find and provide resources. And while a male may benefit from the assistance of his friends, killing a beast can be achieved quite efficiently alone or, at most, with a small group of hunters. Men didn't like to hunt in large packs because then they had to share the spoils. Men who are well adapted to hunt would likely capture more resources and be able to return to the village better able to feed more women and children. He may decide to help the less fortunate with the excess food he has brought back increasing his leadership status within the community. And his skills and ability to acquire more resources may make him feel more confident knowing that he can better fulfill his most important purpose on earth—supporting more children.

The Ashton Kutcher Effect

In 2012, actor and former model Ashton Kutcher, age thirty-three, split from his wife of six years, forty-nine-year-old Demi Moore, following loud public rumors about his infidelity. Since the breakup, Ashton has been linked to many women while sipping champagne around the world.

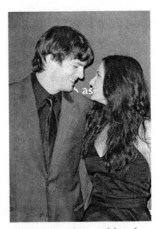

Ashton Kutcher and his then older wife Demi Moore

The powerful evolutionary drive for men to spread their seed and sire many children creates conflicts in modern relationships and society. As mentioned earlier, our goal from an evolutionary perspective is to pass on our genes to the next generation and do our best to find the ideal genetic mate to ensure that our offspring have an even better genetic code. In the not-so-distant past, this meant that a dominant male hunter who could adequately provide for more than one family would be genetically inclined to have more children. At any given time, this genetically fit alpha male's partner could be incapable of bearing more children due to a pregnancy, nursing, or infertility. During those periods, his high levels of testosterone, and likely highly mobile and healthy sperm, would "motivate" him to seek out additional women with which to mate. His first partner would then likely fear losing a portion of her resources to another female and her family. She would be inclined to express feelings of jealousy as an adaptive emotional trait, as well as disdain for the "other woman." She may inform her mate that this woman is unattractive or unsuitable in an attempt to prevent her mate from straying.

> The powerful evolutionary drive for men to spread their seed and sire many children creates conflicts in modern relationships and society.

A woman is evolutionarily driven to protect herself and her offspring's right to the promised resources of the alpha male. Yet, to the highly resourceful and successful alpha male, there is a biological urge driven by evolutionary forces to continue to procreate and it will be difficult to dissuade him.

A male that can provide resources is stamped "beautiful" by nature, and as we discussed earlier, our minds have learned to find attractive or desirable those features that can help us to survive. Attractiveness is a message, this man is likely to be healthy

> Our ancestors who were endowed with a strong chin, brow, and nose had a better chance of survival because they were more protected from fight injuries. To this day, men who possess these dominating masculine traits are found more sexually attractive to women.

and a competent provider. Therefore, from a female's perspective, he likely possesses good genes. However, being resourceful is a dynamic trait that is also heavily influenced by culture and the environment. To be considered resourceful in prehistoric times meant having a strong upper body, a powerful chest, and strong arms, because these features were instrumental for capturing food or defending against predators. Our ancestors who were endowed with a strong chin, brow and nose would also be at an advantage as these bony "faceguards" protected important facial features from fight injuries. Studies have proven that men who possess these dominating masculine traits are found more sexually attractive.(Sadalla, Kenrick & Vershure, 1987).

Physical Characteristics of the Alpha Male

It's no coincidence that the characteristic traits of male dominance are associated with male hormones such as testosterone (Grammer et al., 2003). And humans aren't the only animals with a natural link between dominant physical traits and attractiveness. In fact, throughout the animal kingdom, females prefer male animals that possess the most outstanding traits that help with resourcefulness. The buck with the largest and most symmetric antlers, for example, is most likely to be favored by the female deer and mate earliest in the season. And year after year, the star with the most chiseled features, thick hair, handsome brow, and godly physique is voted the "Sexiest Man Alive" and splashed on the cover of *People* magazine.

Guys learn about the benefits of highly masculine traits during adolescence, when they learn to use their newly acquired physique and express dominance through athletics. This is also when social pecking orders are formed. Although appearance remains a factor as they continue to express their superiority, maturing boys place greater emphasis on, academic achievements, social accomplishments, and political positioning as ways to achieve and express dominance.

> At West Point, freshman cadets with more dominant facial features were more likely to achieve higher rank in the military.

It is not uncommon for the chairman of the board to have the same "prehistoric" characteristics of resourcefulness and be tall, dark, handsome, and physically fit. Perhaps, following years of receiving positive feedback and treatment in school and activities, these physically endowed males learn to expect better treatment, which fuels self-confidence and results in more success. The confidence gained through early successes in physical activity often becomes a self-perpetuating cycle leading to social ascension and success.

There is no denying that when it comes to projecting a favorable first impression, men with the physical traits of strength and resourcefulness gain preference over those less endowed with dominant qualities. And although other signs of resourcefulness are important to a male's projected impression, physical appearance still has a disproportionately great deal of value if pursuing a career in the military, politics or athletics. At the renowned United States Military Academy at West Point, a long-range study revealed that freshman cadets with more dominant facial features defined as broad chins were more likely to achieve higher rank in the military (Muller & Mazur, 1997). The benefits of facial dominance show up in other occupations as well. College males with broad chins are likely to have more girlfriends and more sex (Mazur & Booth, 1998).

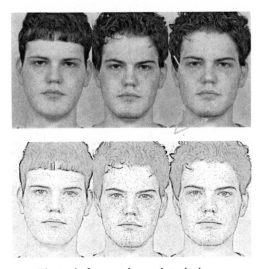

The male face can be made to look more masculine and dominant with an office based filler treatment (Radiesse) to square the cheeks, jaw and chin. Seen with arrows to point out the changes and then in contrast as this makes the alterations more obvious to the conscious mind.

But does a strong chin and wide jaw have anything to do with actual strength?

There is some evolutionary support and reason to believe that better-looking and more masculine-appearing men are indeed stronger and therefore more apt to provide protection to a female. Hands are a quick clue to a man's level of dominance because there is a significant correlation between grip strength, masculinity, facial dominance, and attractiveness (Fink, Neave & Seydel, 2007). And a strong hand with a long ring finger may be especially appealing to a fertile female seeking a mate, because a dominant man can be recognized by his finger size. (Neave, Laing, Fink & Manning, 2003).It appears that testosterone, which leads to a broad chin, cheeks, deep-set eyes, and greater grip strength, also influences finger length during development—it preferentially enlongates the ring finger. In females, higher levels of the sex hormone estrogen create a longer *index* finger than the ring finger. Males with dominant features and higher testosterone levels during fetal develpment can be expected to have a long ring finger, especially in comparison to the index finger. So, for the man with long fingers, there may be value in using his hands when talking—especially if possessing a long ring finger without a ring on it!

When Appearances Don't Deliver

Thirty to fifty something year old men may or may not remember the All American linebacker from The University of Oklahoma, Brian Bosworth? Men like him, a former NFL hopeful, with dominant facial features who doesn't prove to be as good as their genes/appearance advertise, are likely to be more severely punished for their fraud.

When I was in high school, Bosworth was one of my idols. I wanted to be a football star just like him and was convinced I was destined for a career in the NFL. I didn't really pay much attention to academics, had very mediocre grades, and was more captivated by cheerleaders and box scores than books and reading. I wasn't well advised and only applied to four colleges, and when I got rejected from all of them except one, which happened to be too expensive for my family to afford, I felt defeated. I didn't have the heart to tell my hard-working immigrant father or disabled mother my failure. Fortunately, I was invited to meet with the football coach of a small, highly respected, private Midwestern University to assess my interest in playing football. It was by no means a powerhouse Division One or Big Ten School, but it provided "relaxed standards" for accepting student athletes. I was lucky to get in, and fortunately my situation allowed me to qualify for a large financial aid package to help with the very expensive tuition. I decided to enroll, but when I told my high school counselors they strongly urged me to not attend. They said it was too academic and advanced for me. All I could say was, "But I want be a doctor one day. I have to go there."

> Attractive men who shatter the image of the admirable, protective alpha male are often brutally reviled for defaming that image.

My counselors recommended I go to community college for the summer to prepare, but that wasn't going to happen because I was way too motivated to have a fun summer. After that, it was clear that I was going to have my work cut out for me if I was to tackle a pre-med curriculum.

When I got to college, I realized that as a five-foot-nine wide receiver who ran a four-point-nine forty-yard dash, my livelihood wasn't going to be made in the NFL. I figured I'd be better off studying chemistry and biology then doing push-ups and sprints, so I gave up my dream and studied and studied and studied. I became incredibly driven to do well in school and developed an insatiable appetite for knowledge. I missed my gridiron days, but my football icons faded as I began to admire people like Einstein, Freud, and Franklin. I wasn't destined to become Brian Bosworth, and that was all right because I found my real passion could be achieved through a career in medicine.

What happened to Bosworth? Well he was drafted first round and turned out to be a bust, not the superstar everyone predicted. I remember him getting run over by former Heisman Trophy winner and superstar running back Bo Jackson in a Monday Night Football game, which marked Bosworth as a lamb. He quickly fell out of favor and was brutally reviled and defamed. I don't mean to pick on Brian Bosworth—every year there's a handful of first-round draft choices in all sports who don't turn out to be what we want them to be, and who are then subjected to harsh verbal punishment. We react almost as if they fooled and cheated us by advertising promise and then not delivering. The disappointment and resentment that comes from feeling duped by external appearances results in highly touted athletes receiving disproportionally severe ridicule and often becoming the butt of jokes for years.

A similar phenomenon happens to men who are particularly attractive, but use their good looks to swindle or take advantage of the less fortunate. In legal proceedings, attractive men are more likely to be found guilty and severely penalized in cases of rape or murder. Sensational media attention surrounded the cases of Robert Chambers, known as the "Preppie Killer," Scott Peterson and Joran van der Sloot—all handsome, well-to-do men who murdered women and shattered the image of the admirable, protective alpha male.

Handsome Is Electable

Dominant physical traits matter in politics and elections. In 2010, conservative Scott Brown won the election for U.S. Senator from the very liberal state of Massachusetts. In addition to being a moderate Republican, Brown happens to be a tall, attractive man with a full head of hair and dominant physical traits. In fact, about thirty years before he won his senate seat he posed for a centerfold in *Cosmopolitan Magazine*.

> In presidential campaigns, the candidate with the more dominant male facial features is more likely to win the election.

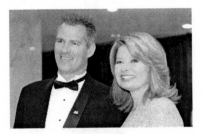

Scott Brown was a model in his younger years.

His fellow New Englander, Mitt Romney, a former governor, successful businessman and Republican candidate for the 2012 presidential nomination, is also an attractive, "Ken doll" type. And our tall, handsome, well-proportioned and athletic President commands an audience when he swaggers into a room. Is it a coincidence that our male leaders are attractive? Not at all.

As much as we want to believe we don't consider physical appearance when electing our leaders, we often do. The better-looking male candidate often wins the election (Hamermesh, 2006). In an unpublished study I conducted in 2008, we measured the forehead slope, chin position, and jaw width of all the U.S. presidential candidates of the television age, from Kennedy/Nixon to Bush/Kerry. We found that the candidate with the more dominant male facial features was more likely to win the election.

And, if you think we could actually be that shallow when picking the winner of a race, a study conducted by investigators at Princeton asked over 600 people to judge photographs of candidates running for Congress in the 2000, 2002, and 2004 elections (Todorov, Mandisodza, Goren & Hall, 2005). The volunteers didn't know about the candidates' political viewpoints, but were asked to judge them on competency and other traits such as honesty, trustworthiness, leadership, charisma, intelligence, and likability. More than any other trait, the candidate's perceived competency clinched his electability. The more competent-appearing candidate won the election seventy percent of the time. Even when volunteers were given just one second to view the photo and make a judgment, they came to the same conclusion. The candidates rated as more competent by their appearance alone were more likely to win.

In comments about this study, Leslie Zebrowitz from Brandeis University noted that baby-faced individuals, characterized by having a round face, large eyes, small nose, large forehead, and small chin, were perceived as less competent. Why? Once again, this perception has been ingrained in our subconscious mind. A childlike-looking person suggests someone who is naïve, submissive and weak, and therefore likely to be less competent and less able to lead. So, while infantile features are important in advertising, we don't want our elected leaders to be baby-faced.

Save the Smile

Interestingly, we don't want our men to be too friendly looking, either. We conducted a study on first impressions in which we asked volunteers to rate their first impressions of people who were either smiling or with a neutral expression (Dayan et al., 2008). We found that those individuals with big, large smiles with teeth showing were perceived as less trustworthy. This confused me. It didn't seem right, but I am not the only one who has noted the disadvantages a wide smile can have on one's projected impression. Sociologist Allan Mazur showed that men with a big, wide smile are actually perceived as having less facial dominance. Furthermore, it turns out that men who smile more broadly are less likely to achieve a higher rank and status in the military (Mazur, Mazur & Keating, 1984).

Men with big, toothy smiles are seen as less trustworthy or dominant.

One look at CEO walls of fame in corporate headquarters or photos of our U.S. presidents reveals that these highly respected and dominant men rarely wear a broad smile. A hint of friendliness is welcome, but we don't associate a wide, open grin with a powerful leader. So, men who want to project an image of being in charge in order to get a job or look powerful on his Facebook page would improve their chances with a photo in which they don't wear a broad smile. Save the big smile for the trip to Disney with the kids.

Historically, height was also an important dominance factor for our prehistoric relatives because it gave them a vantage point over the terrain granting them an edge in both fighting and retrieving food. And today, we still prefer height in our leaders. All the U.S. presidents except James Madison and Benjamin Harrison were of above-average height for their time. Furthermore, in all the presidential elections, the taller candidate won except twice: Nixon over McGovern and Bush over Kerry. In his 2005 bestseller *Blink*, Malcolm Gladwell revealed that thirty percent of Fortune 500 CEOs were above six-foot-two compared to only four percent of the normal population.

Additionally, a business school study revealed that taller men were more likely to be hired for a higher salary (Frieze, Olson & Good, 1990).

Studies also show that taller men are thought to be more athletic, attractive, physically fit, and have a higher professional status. Women prefer sperm donors who are taller men, and in a 2008 *USA Today* poll of active and retired CEOs and other leading executives, ninety-five percent of respondents said that if given a choice, they would rather be bald than short (Jones, 2008). And of the thirty-one CEOs who said they were bald or balding, all agreed that being short was more detrimental to moving up in an executive career than baldness.

This might be why growth hormone is one of the most misused drugs in America today. Growth hormone, a natural substance in everyone's body, is released from the pituitary gland and regulates many functions, including bone growth. Some people suffer from diseases caused by excessive growth hormone, such as acromegaly or

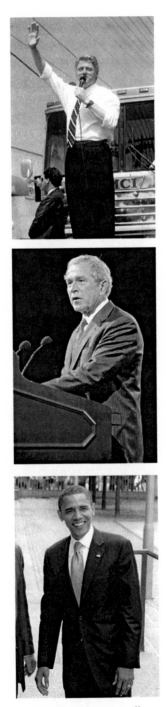

Presidents are generally taller than average.

gigantism, which makes them very tall with enormous jaws, thick brows, and large hands and feet. These traits produce an aggressive appearance and often instill fear in others. The movie actor Richard Kiel who played the metal-toothed "Jaws" in the 1970s James Bond movies and the famed WWF wrestler Andre the Giant are two famous examples of men who capitalized on this rare condition.

> The taller hunter on the plains had the advantage, and today the taller candidate usually wins and the taller applicant gets hired at a higher salary. It's no surprise that most men would rather be bald than short.

At the other end of the spectrum, people who are deficient in growth hormone are unusually short and don't mature normally. An estimated one in 3,500 children in the U.S. are growth hormone deficient, and for them, taking growth hormone is very important to achieving a normal life. But there is a rising rate of abuse of the hormone in the United States as parents seek it out for their kids who they think might be falling short of their desired height. Many socially and economically successful parents who want their kids to have an advantage in the world are pushing their pediatricians to give them growth hormone. Whether it is the five-foot-four father who believes his child will be better off in business if he reaches a height of five-foot-eight or the parent of the star varsity quarterback who, at only five-ten, is likely to be overlooked for that big college scholarship unless he reaches a height of at least six-two.

Misusing growth hormone to gain height and potential advantage later in life is becoming commonplace. Although the risks of serious side effects are substantial (Rosenbloom & Rivkees, 2010) and the price tag very high at 1,000 to 3,000 dollars per month, many well-meaning parents see this as a worthy investment that is sure to pay off for their child years later.

This desire for additional height isn't unique to Western culture. In China, where the average male height is five-foot-six and average female height five-foot-two, there's a trend to increase height in order to compete with the West. As a result, dangerous surgery to lengthen the leg bones has become popular, but remains very controversial. In fact, it was outlawed in 2006, but reports show that it is still being performed.

There are safe and effective options for men who are not naturally endowed with height, standing with an erect posture, being physically fit, and wearing form-fitting clothing can all make a dramatic difference and project a strong, confident image consistent with height.

The Walking, Talking Gene Ad

Brad Pitt was gifted with a full set of ideal traits that add up to extreme male attractiveness: a tall stature, V-shaped chest, heavy brows, deep-set eyes, symmetrical nose, projecting

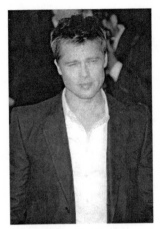

Brad Pitt. Nothing else needs to be said.

chin, and a wide, angular jaw. Appearing tall, masculine, symmetric, and powerful is vital to attracting the most desirable mate. These qualities that we throw together in the term "good-looking" are all subconscious clues indicating health, vitality and good genes, and there is evidence that facial attractiveness may be correlated to better quality semen (Soler et al., 2003).

Women following their instinctive drive to find ideal genes from quality sperm can't help but be attracted to symmetric-appearing dominant males. Through eons of time, women have learned that a male's facial appearance may very well match up with better quality semen and thus better offspring. And what's even more interesting is that a female's attraction to the well-endowed, genetically fit male is even stronger when she is in her fertile ovulatory phase of her menstrual cycle.

My cousin, whom I introduced earlier, is extremely good looking, tall, dark, athletic, intelligent and financially well off. He's the complete package and very eligible, but also a serial dater who has not yet met the woman who can tame him. To many men he lives the dream. He likes to date multiple women at a time and has a somewhat checkered reputation among many of Chicago's top females. They know he's trouble and want to stand clear and avoid him if he's nearby, but like gawkers who can't help sneaking a peek at a car wreck, many well-to-do, eligible women can't resist being attracted to his powerful image. Most recently, I gave this warning to a young woman in her early thirties, recently divorced with one child

> The subconscious urges of the female body and mind know when the time is right for an encounter with the powerful genes and sperm of a strong, genetically well-endowed male.

and strikingly beautiful. Knowing that my single cousin would not likely be interested in a serious or long-term relationship with her, I advised her to stay away from him if she was looking for something more deep and lasting. However, the more we told her to stay away the more interested she seemed to become. It was as if they were both being challenged to not fall for each other.

> A strong chin is associated with masculinity, strength, and vitality, and for men who don't have one, the cheapest and easiest way to achieve the same effect is to grow out their facial hair.

And, true to his form, once my cousin found his prey he circled her, cased her out and, when the timing was just right, went in for the kill. They dated for about four months. They enjoyed each other's company, but everyone assumed it wasn't going to go very far—including both of them—and it didn't. I don't think either is worse off for it; they both seemed to be content with a short-term romantic game plan.

Both men and women are wired for short- and long-term mating strategies that work on a subconscious level and are driven by biological desires. In the short-term, a woman wants the most physically dominating male with the strongest genetic features; however, that same female's long-term strategies are more focused on finding a male that will be loyal, stay close to home, and provide continuous resources for growing offspring. And when a woman is in the fertile portion of her menstrual cycle, her desire steers her toward the more genetically fit male. She becomes particularly attracted to hyper-masculine, dominant appearing males—the Brad Pitt type. This is why women are more likely to have affairs and sexual fantasies about dominant-appearing men when they are in the fertile portion of their cycle and why dominant, highly symmetric men are most likely to have more sexual encounters. The subconscious urges of the female body and mind know when the time is right for an encounter with the powerful genes and sperm of a strong, genetically well-endowed male (Bellis & Baker, 1990; Gangestad & Cousins, 2001; Gangestad, Simpson, Cousins, Garver-Apgar & Christensen, 2004; S. W. Gangestad, Thornhill & Garver, 2002; Jones et al., 2005; Mazur et al., 1984).

Today, men who are not blessed with naturally dominant facial features such as a prominent jawline or chin have medical options at their disposal to create these features with both permanent and non-permanent synthetic implants. Prior to modern-day plastic surgery, options for the mandible-challenged male were far and few between. It's rumored that when George Washington stood for his portrait he placed cotton in his mouth to expand his chin and jawline, evidently recognizing that a strong, broad chin represented leadership qualities.

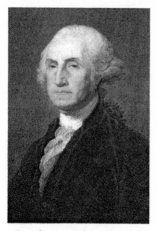

Our first president knew the importance of appearing masculine and strong.

For those turned off by cottonmouth or unable to afford either the time or expense of a medical treatment, there is a proven traditional method for highlighting and enhancing male facial features. Even better, it doesn't cost a dime and is 100 percent effective. The best way for a man to accentuate his masculine features is to grow out his facial hair. This is the reason many women seem to like a man with a little bit of stubble on the chin and jaw. Many men with small or weak chins not in proportion with the rest of their face wear goatees and beards to override those features. A small chin is a feminine feature, whereas a strong chin is associated with masculinity, strength, and vitality.

With their rock-solid and shelf-like jawlines, superheroes such as Batman, Superman, and Iron Man all seem to be blessed with galactic levels of testosterone. Contrast this with Andy Gump, the famous chinless and cowardly depression-era cartoon character or the popular ninety-eight-pound weakling in the 1930 Charles Atlas cartoons who acquiesces to getting sand kicked in his face. A beard or goatee will accentuate the chin and mitigate an image of weakness. Knowing this, it isn't surprising that many of the men who come to me requesting a chin implant walk in the office sporting a goatee. After surgery, donning a new masculine-projecting chin, they never seem to grow the goatee again. I don't think these men consciously choose to grow a goatee to accommodate for a weak chin, but they are prewired like the rest of us to realize that a small chin represents weakness and needs to be built up.

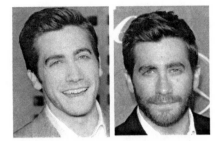

When sporting a fuller beard, actor Jake Gyllenhaal shows how facial hair adds width to a man's face and strengthens the appearance of his chin, both of which are traits of male facial dominance.

Tall, Dark and Handsome vs. Short, Red and Boyish

"Along with the ninety-seven percent of women who can see, I have never been a fan of redheaded men," declared talk-show host, comedian and author Chelsea Handler.

Across all populations and cultures, we like men to be darker than women. Regardless of geography, males are consistently a bit darker in complexion than females. Felt to be a sexually dimorphic trait, females are designed to be paler so that they absorb more

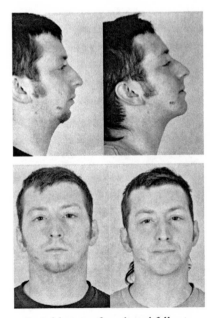

Facial hair is often shaved following chin implant surgery.

sunlight because they need vitamin D for their bones and during childbearing, as mentioned earlier (Russell, 2003). In contrast, males need to be darker to protect them from excessive sun exposure while out hunting. Therefore, males are perceived as more attractive when their skin and hair color are a few shades darker than their female counterparts. For this reason, we prefer tall, dark and handsome over short, red and light.

Studies show that redheaded men have a disadvantage because women really do discriminate against them. In one study, redheaded males were determined to be less attractive, less intelligent, less masculine, and less successful. This stereotype seems to be strong and consistent, at least among Anglos (Clayson & Maughn, 1976). Moreover, Cryos, one of the world's largest sperm banks, is no longer accepting donations from redheaded males because of low preference for this sperm (Orange, 2011). Of course, like any rule, there are exceptions. The incredibly smart, successful, and pale redhead Conan O'Brien is doing just fine, for example. However, if you are a redheaded man who wants to be the leader of the pack and you feel that you're being unfairly discriminated against, you may want to consider darkening your hair.

Does Size Really Matter?

In the many parts of the world I traveled while researching this book, Southeast Asia, and Cambodia in particular, stand out in my memory. I was struck by one detail of the ancient architecture in the region of Angkor Wat in the deep south of Cambodia, a region famous for its temples which date back to the twelfth century.

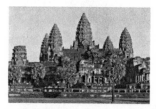

Angkor Wat in Cambodia

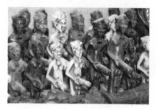

*Amulets to gods
with large penises*

I was fascinated and inspired by these sites with their distinctive towers that penetrate deep into the sky. Rounded at the top, these structures look like large penises. And the worship of the erect penis is not just limited to the temples; I saw amulets and other small objects for wearing or placing in the home that were shaped like erect penises. There was no hiding the erect penis as an object of worship.

I was startled by this at first, but on further thought I realized that the Khmer people aren't much different from the ancient Egyptians who build obelisks to their gods, Hindus who worshipped a god in a phallic form known as the Lingam, Europeans who designed steeples in their cathedrals and Americans who created the Washington monument. The fascination with phallic symbols can be found everywhere. The male penis has been deified from the ancient Egyptian god, Min, to the Greek god, Priapus.

Modern architecture takes the obsession to the extreme with a constant race for the tallest skyscraper. Growing up in Chicago, we were so proud of our Sears Tower, which for twenty-five years was the tallest building in the world. It's still the tallest in the United States, but now that distinction goes to Burj Khalifa in Dubai. A 160-story building plunging into the sky is pretty impressive, but when it comes to men and their penises, does size really matter?

Let's get this question out of the way since it's a big issue for men who insist on arguing, posturing, and referring to the size of their male-defining appendage. From musicians to athletes, genital gestures for males are a way to strut their manliness.

Just like the nose is important to facial beauty because of its relation to the midline, the penis is a midline structure that can be a source of anxiety to many males. As many as ten percent of males who visit an obsessive-compulsive disorder clinic are overly concerned with their

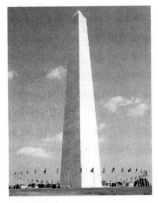

The Washington monument

penises (Phillips & Diaz, 1997). Although most females don't give it the same interest, males may become fixated on penis position and size. But how much do females care about the appearance of a penis?

Much like female genitalia, the penis is rarely described as attractive or ugly. By the time they get to the penis, most females have already decided whether or not they are going to engage based on many other physical and emotional clues. In a large survey of over 25,000 sexually active heterosexual women between the ages of eighteen to sixty-five, eighty-five percent said they were satisfied with their partner's penis size, fourteen percent wanted their partner to be larger and two percent wanted their partner to be smaller (Lever, Frederick & Peplau, 2006). This data is consistent with another survey in which the majority of sexually active females didn't think the size of the penis was important; however, when asked further about the importance of the penis' dimensions, twenty-one percent found the length of the penis to be most important and thirty-three percent found the girth to be most important, suggesting that thickness of the penis is more important than length (Francken, van de Wiel, van Driel & Weijmar Schultz, 2002).

> In spite of the way many men obsess over it, the majority of sexually active women don't think penis size is important.

With men, it's a different story. In a large survey of over 25,000 males, only 55 percent were satisfied with their penis size. Of those men who said their penis size was of average size, over forty percent desired to have a bigger penis. Interestingly, the satisfaction most men had with their penis size correlated with their self-perception or satisfaction they have with their face and body. Generally speaking, men who are happy with their penis size also are confident in their appearance (Lever, et al., 2006). For the record, the average size of the erect penis has been calculated to be 5.3 inches with 68 percent of men measuring between 4.6 and 6.0 inches, 13.5 percent between 3.8 and 4.5 inches and 13.5

percent between 6.1 and 6.8 inches. Only about 2.5 percent of men surveyed had a penis over 6.9 inches long and 2.5 percent were less than 3.7 inches long (Lever, et al., 2006).

So, are men overly concerned about their male appendage size, or are females underreporting its importance? Masters and Johnson concluded that size really didn't matter to female sexual satisfaction because they noted that the vagina will adapt to any size penis (Masters & Johnson, 2010). Why then do men strut their dominance by emphasizing their manliness? Is there some evolutionary significance and importance to the shape and size of the male penis?

> If the penis has evolved to be a weapon of sperm-placing dominance between males, it makes sense that men would feel competitive about their penis size.

The human penis is proportionally much larger than those of our primate cousins, the ape and chimpanzee. The larger glans, head and coronal ridge (the leading edge around the head) may have evolved as a "seminal displacement" device. This means that a larger penis with a bigger head may be more efficient at scooping out the semen of another man from a female vagina and winning the sperm competition to fertilize the egg (Gallup et al., 2003). This theory, published in 2002, is the result of a study performed at the State University of New York (SUNY), which included mechanical testing with model vaginas and penises designed to measure the ability of a latex mechanical penis to displace fluid from the vaginal canal. They noted that the unique design of the penis displaces fluid and washes it behind the coronal ridge, sending it to the outside of the vaginal canal. Additionally, the deeper the thrust, the more effective the penis was at displacing the fluid.

Their study was followed up with a behavioral survey of 295 college students from SUNY in Albany, which further supported the theory that the shape of the penis is a design that evolved to win the sperm competition. In their survey, both males and females reported that sexual intercourse, performed after suspecting their partner of infidelity, was characterized with faster and deeper thrusting. This inferred that if a man was suspicious that his partner was with another man, he would want to work harder sexually to displace another man's semen and win the competition to fertilize the egg. So, if the penis has evolved to be a weapon of dominance between males, it makes sense that men would feel competitive about their penis size.

As for women, a larger, thicker penis should therefore indicate that a man is more genetically favorable, and it would follow that women would instinctively be interested in a larger penis. But surveys don't bear that out. Surveys aren't hugely reliable, though, because there's nothing preventing women from being biased in their responses. It's possible that they've been educated to *say* that size doesn't matter, while on some level they feel that it actually does.

One group of researchers took a more solid approach to find out if penis size matters to women. In that study, women were shown a series of photos of naked men in which the only variation was the size of the penis. The four sizes shown were 78%, 122%, 133% or 143% of normal, but the women were not told that the penis size was altered. In the photos they found most attractive, the penis size was 133% of normal, not 143%. Hmm . . . so a bit bigger is nice, but not too big (Dixson, Dixson, Li & Anderson, 2007).

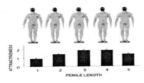

The slightly larger penis at 133% of normal was preferred. (Dixson, Am J Hum Biol, 19(1), 88-95 2007)

The Ups and Downs of Testosterone

Just as a too-large penis isn't considered attractive, too much testosterone also turns women away. For example, an excessively broad chin, heavy brow, or darkened eyes represent male features that signal a man who is aggressive, dominant, unfriendly, threatening, volatile, controlling, manipulative, coercive, and selfish (Grammer, Fink, Møller & Thornhill, 2003). A woman's negative response to these traits is likely due to the fact that these facial characteristics are produced by high testosterone levels during development, making it an evolutionary adaptive trait that matches higher testosterones levels with possible aggressiveness (Dabbs, Jurkovic & Frady, 1991). Fear-provoking faces may be great in horror movies, but because females rely on stable relationships for their offspring to survive, a first impression that indicates too much male aggressiveness works against a man (Grammer et al., 2003). Over millions of years of evolution, females have learned to fear these individuals.

Because women rely on stable relationships for their offspring to survive, a first impression that indicates too much male aggressiveness works against a man.

I treat a male patient who, unfortunately, possesses these over-aggressive-looking traits. He is constantly trying to soften his features and tells me that he is perceived as mean or angry, when in actuality he is not.

For men with excessive male-defining characteristics, overly aggressive facial features can severely detract from their success in business or mating. Our amygdala, one of the most primitive portions of our brain, is prewired to fear these character traits. Science has shown that men with higher levels of testosterone are linked with dominance and competition, and although the finding is controversial, their excess hormone levels may even be associated

Today, women in Western society value male socioeconomic status, wealth, and social prestige more than male physical attractiveness.

with violent behavior (Studer, Aylwin & Reddon, 2005). However, while excess testosterone may be found in criminals, it cannot be said to be a risk factor or cause of criminality. Criminal behavior is based on several factors, but undoubtedly testosterone levels may be reliably associated with excessive competitiveness or risky behaviors.

Excessive or otherwise, brawn may be on the way out.

In a modern civilization, the value of testosterone in developing physical signs of dominance has diminished as resourcefulness has shifted away from muscles and a powerful physique to more modern character traits needed for success. However, here again we see testosterone linked to competition in financial, political, or social status (Mazur & Booth, 1998). It's likely that if you were to test the testosterone levels of Wall Street or corporate boardroom executives, their levels would be higher than their more subdued, couch-potato contemporaries. In civilized Western society, signs of resourcefulness today are as contingent on social, political and financial prowess as muscles and physical strength were for millions of years prior.

> Women at their height of fertility—when ovulating—prefer a more dominating male appearance, but when they are not ovulating they desire a man who is less masculine and more feminine appearing.

Today, women in Western society value male socioeconomic status, wealth, and social prestige more than male physical attractiveness (Grammer et al., 2003). Women still seek out the most resourceful male for the same reasons, but the clues to resourcefulness they're looking for has taken on a whole new form. Both men and women are aware of this, and that's why male professional status is so highly valued and competed for by testosterone-fueled men. Men intuitively know what women are seeking in a mate, and the man who is less physically endowed can make up for what he lacks in looks by the size of his wallet. Women prefer average or even unattractive men with lucrative occupations to attractive men with low status professions (Townsend & Levy, 1990).

So, when a woman is at her sexual peak and interested in finding a sexual partner she will likely be attracted to a male with evidence of high but not excessive levels of testosterone. Such a male likely has physical signs of strength and vitality which clues in the female that he is a holder of good sperm. However, somewhat strangely, this same male is not someone from whom a female desires monogamy. She rather prefers a male with lower levels of the testosterone. Interestingly, when males get married or are in a committed relationship, their testosterone levels drop! They are no longer on the hunt and they need to stay home and take care of the offspring. Testosterone fires up libido, and men who are married or committed don't need such a strong sex drive (Wang et al., 2000). Accordingly, males with lower levels of testosterone are shown to be more faithful to their spouses. They also have better immunity and are less likely to enter risky behavior, both of which combine to make them more likely to survive and be a provider for offspring (Burnham et al., 2003).

Excess levels of testosterone have been shown to reduce immunity and be associated with risky or aggressive behaviors (Starzyk & Quinsey, 2001) and even earlier death. For these reasons, a female will adjust the type of male she finds attractive based on her menstrual cycle. Women at their height of fertility—when ovulating—prefer a more dominating male appearance, but when they are not ovulating they desire a man who is less masculine and more feminine appearing (Johnston, Hagel, Franklin, Fink & Grammer, 2001; Penton-Voak et al., 1999).

> As important as a man's dominating physical appearance may be for the short-term, women place more importance on factors such as intelligence and social status when looking for a longer-term mate.

As important as a man's dominating physical appearance may be for the short-term, women place more importance on factors such as intelligence and social status when looking for a longer-term mate (Prokosch, Cossa, Scheib & Blozisa, 2009). Ultimately, a woman desires protection and resourcefulness from a mate. And for men more financially endowed, this means more chances to mate with beautiful females corroborating Aristotle Onassis' thoughts on money: "All the money in the world would make no difference if women didn't exist."

All of this explains why single males dripping with testosterone and prowling for mates parade with loud jewelry, branded clothing, and expensive cars. They want to call attention to the wealth/resourcefulness that they know is powerfully attractive to the opposite sex. It's also why the salt-and-pepper George Clooney appeals to younger women. A mature male is more attractive because he has had time to acquire more resources then younger men. The male with resources also inherently realizes that he can trade in these resources for a female with valued physical assets. This perhaps explains why young and beautiful "trophy wives" are found on the arms of wealthy, successful businessmen—and why the average age difference between such a man and his first wife is just under three years, between a second wife five years and a third wife eight years. At the extreme end of this phenomenon, Hugh Hefner, at eighty years of age, can have three girlfriends.

However, men who want to appear resourceful have to keep in mind that if they overdo their showmanship, it will have the opposite effect. Just like the overly tan female with too much makeup or excess collagen in her lips will turn away males, wearing gaudy fake jewelry or overtly acting rich will tip off females that the man is a fraud and not genuinely resourceful.

Perhaps this explains Henry Kissinger's famous line when referring to men, "Power is the greatest aphrodisiac." However, the opposite is not true—men place little value on a woman's occupation when assessing her attractiveness (Grammar, 2003; Townsend, 1990).

The competition for the ideal mate is fierce on both sides. Women compete for men by trying to one-up each other in appearance, while men work just as vigorously to appear more resourceful than the other guy. When couples go out to dinner, the men often engage in conversation with the men and women with the women because male and female interests are invariably very different from each other. To a great extent, what each gender finds important is largely based on their prewired biological drives. If you understand these basic evolutionary forces, the context of the conversations seems to make more sense.

What's more difficult to live and unfortunately undeniable is the anti-monogamous streak that runs deep in both male and female biology. While monogamy for a period of time is important to the human species' genetic survival because it allows offspring to be better equipped to live and thrive, for some males and females with a particular genetic makeup, serial monogamy (finding a new mate once the offspring are self-sufficient) may be more adaptive and preferred by Mother Nature than staying with one long-term mate.

While discomforting to hear, with both men and women programmed for "genetic immortality," it's not easy to conform to the moral and civil expectations of our times. Nature designs genetically successful women to seek out a certain kind of man when she's most fertile, yet desire another type when she's not. And well-endowed men are driven by a powerful drive to spread their seed as far and wide as possible as long as they can provide. Nature has its reasons, but it almost seems cruel! A review of more than forty years of research on infidelity reveals that the likelihood of cheating during the course of a marriage runs from thirty to sixty percent for men and twenty to fifty percent for women (Buss & Shackelford, 1997). Once we know the underlying—and awkwardly natural—sources of this behavior, we may have better insight into each other and how to prevent it.

As we continue to make our first steps into modern civilization during our long journey as human beings, maybe some of our strongest moral priorities, like monogamy, will start to have an impact on our evolution. We may be destined to move further and further away from our primal drives. But then again, with millions of years of survival-tested evolution still laser focused on producing good genes . . . maybe not.

CHAPTER 5

SCENTS AND SENSIBILITY

"When women are in the presence of a preferred scent, they are more likely to project positive feelings on those around them, which can lead to increased attraction."

—Dr. Alan Hirsch

There's more to first impressions than meets the eye. Have you ever been out with a couple of friends when a stunning guy or woman walked your way, but you quickly lost interest? At first, this god-like creature looked extremely attractive, but as he or she got closer, you lost the spark. By the time the person passed by, you barely even noticed them. You may have even looked away, but your friends were still captivated. Why were you turned off but your friends so turned on?

It wasn't your vision. It was your nose.

Your indifference or even distaste was probably due to that person's odor—and I'm not talking about Chanel No. 5 or Armani. You picked up that person's raw, unique, natural, and identifying smell. For each of us, that scent is a silent calling signal that lies at the heart of nature's sexual and mating strategy. Even though we're unaware of it, our individual scent is critical to our attractiveness and choosing a mate. For many years, scientists, knowing full well the necessity of scent in the animal kingdom, were quick to discount its value in humans. But when the facts started coming in, boy, were we surprised.

Chemical messengers called pheromones appear to be one of the most important ingredients in choosing and keeping a mate. The term pheromone comes from the Greek words *pherein* (to carry) and *hormone* (to excite), and science is well aware of their crucial role in the animal kingdom. Emitted from the body into the environment, they activate specific physiological or psychological responses in other individuals of the same species(Grammer, Fink & Neave, 2005).

Scientists have also learned a lot about the power of human pheromones. The chemical identity of our pheromones is unique to each individual, much like a fingerprint. We have a set of genes that code for proteins that are individual to each person and are embedded in every cell of the body, known as the major histocompatibility complex (MHC). Our MHC gives our immune system the ability to detect whether a cell is our own or a foreign invader. You may share comparable MHC with your relatives (MHC-similar), but two unrelated people are very unlikely to have the same or similar MHC (MHC-dissimilar).

MHC is a serious factor when looking for a match for organ transplant surgery. Blood samples are carefully analyzed to find the ideal match—the more similar the MHC, the more likely the patient will accept the other person's organ. Identical twins have the exact same MHC and relatives are MHC-similar, but the further two people are separated by geography and population, the more dissimilar their MHC. The MHC of someone from Western Africa, for example, would be very different than that of someone from Eastern Europe.

Our MHC provides a code that relates to our immunity and our pheromones. Our pheromones are a calling card of our immunity and identity, and people whose MHC is made up of a complex mix of different codes possess what's known as a distinct heterozygous MHC. This type is associated with a more genetically fit person who is likely to carry more symmetric features and be physically beautiful. As discussed earlier, natural selection prefers the highly mixed gene complex because a person with that kind of genetic code is more equipped to deal with a wide variety of stresses from the environment. The more complex the code, the more tools the body can draw upon for survival when a germ or other threat comes its way. A simpler genetic code doesn't give the body as many options.

> A person with a highly mixed gene complex is more equipped to deal with a wide variety of stresses from the environment.

To illustrate this, imagine you're on a trek with your best friend in a remote, rocky wilderness where the weather is wildly variable, ranging from extreme heat to icy cold and desert-dry to sopping wet. You're wearing the latest in protective outdoor clothing, with multiple layers that can repel water and absorb moisture, block the wind when zipped, or allow a cooling breeze to flow in when it's hot. Your shoes are water-resistant, supportive, and very comfortable. Your friend, on the other hand, sports an old sweatshirt, sweatpants, and a pair of flip-flops. Before long he's been battered by the weather and needs time to rest and tend to his cut and blistered feet. While his simple, one-layer outfit makes him susceptible to all the changing elements, you're equipped to pull on or peel off layers as you need them.

In your ready-for-anything outfit, you're like the person with a varied gene complex who is better equipped to tolerate extremes. Local parasites, bacteria and viruses adapt to an environment and tend to take advantage of the genetic common denominators within a population. People with a highly differentiated gene complex tend to code for different proteins that can help them become resistant to many kinds of "bugs." These people are more likely to survive, thrive, and pass on their genes through multiple offspring. This is evolution's process of adaptation, so when it comes to finding an ideal mate, nature says, "Similar MHC bad—dissimilar MHC good!"

But how do we know *who* has the most genetically fit and well-endowed code in their cells? Nature tells us by displaying a strong genetic code through physical traits such as facial symmetry, averageness, clear skin, and a full head of hair, which are just a few of the signs. Collectively, however, we just recognize these traits as beautiful. And males and females with greater symmetry, the appropriate waist-to-hip ratios, and prettier hair, skin and eyes tend to possess good genes *and* smell pleasant to the opposite sex (Gangestad & Thornhill, 1998; Oberzaucher & Grammer, 2009).

> The MHC imprinted in your personal scent is like an aromatic billboard that advertises your genetic makeup and fertility.

The MHC imprinted in your personal scent is like an aromatic billboard, "seen" through your nose, which advertises your genetic makeup and fertility.

There's Beauty in the Air

To test the idea that there may be a connection between beauty and the scent a woman emits researchers asked a group of men to look at photographs of women and rate their attractiveness. They asked another group of men to smell the t-shirts these same women slept in for three nights and describe the scent. Guess what? The women whom the first group rated most attractive were the same women who the second group rated their t-shirt odors as sexy, erotic, and pleasant. The study concluded that beauty seems to be communicated by pheromones because beautiful women emit sexy odors (Rikowski & Grammer, 1999).

In *Scent of a Woman*, Al Pacino's Academy Award-winning performance as the blind Lieutenant Colonel Frank Slade intoxicated us with the sensual effects of smell: "Ooh, but I still smell her. Women! What can you say? Who made 'em? . . . The hair . . . they say the hair is everything, you know. Have you ever buried your nose in a mountain of curls . . . just wanted to go to sleep forever?"

Research backs up that a blind person like Col. Slade could indeed identify an attractive person based on his or her smell alone! And the information stored in our MHC also tells much more. Like nature's Facebook, MHC makes public some of the details about our identity and social status, and also reveals if we are fertile, ovulating, ready to mate, or not interested.

> Like nature's Facebook, MHC makes public some of the details about our identity and social status, and also reveals if we are fertile, ovulating, ready to mate, or not interested.

We secrete pheromones from glands around the armpits, genitals, and anus, right next to sweat glands that release fatty acids and proteins that attract bacteria. It's the bacteria in these areas, not the pheromones themselves, which are responsible for what we call "B.O." Just watch two dogs when they meet each other for the first time. Where do they immediately go to get acquainted? They head for the pheromones, which happen to be in an area that carries some other smells as well.

In the animal world, ovulating females secrete strong pheromones that serve as a calling signal that they are ready to mate. Males pick up the signal and get ready to copulate. Without the presence of pheromones, males are much less interested in sex. But humans are the big exception— we may be the only species that will spend valuable energy and resources on sex without the intent of getting the female pregnant. Although we are starting to learn there may be more sex for pleasure in the animal kingdom than we once thought; males of most non-human species don't want to waste their time chasing females just to have sex with them if it's not going to result in fertilization.

> Women release odors that tell men they are fertile and ready to mate.

They wait for external cues such as swelling genitalia that show that a female is in "heat," or ovulating, *and* the presence of pheromones. Female monkeys let the males know they are ready by releasing fatty acids called copulins into the air from the vagina. The smells within these copulins alert males that a female is ovulating.

Do human females do the same thing? Studies show that yes, women release odors from their vaginas that announce they are fertile and ready to mate. Human males who were exposed to copulins and then asked to rate the attractiveness of female photos said that the odor didn't smell particularly pleasant, but rated females more attractive after taking a whiff (Kirk-Smith, Booth, Carroll, & Davies, 1978). It is believed that the copulins secreted from a female's pubic area are detected by an organ at the base of the nose called the vomeronasal organ (VNO). This area picks up the pheromone and sends a signal to primitive portions of the brain to recognize that the woman is ovulating and results in increased blood flow to the man's genitalia.

All of this happens subconsciously as the chemicals respond to each other and trigger physical changes. Additionally, the man becomes overwhelmed with the idea of mating in light of a ripe, fertile, and friendly woman and places less emphasis on factors like facial beauty, which is normally a very important indicator of health and vitality.

So, for the opportunistic man on the hunt for a mate, a woman's facial appearance takes a back seat to her "ready-to-go" signaling copulins. This may be one of the reasons Arnold "the Governator" slept with his house staffer who was close by and easy prey instead of spending the energy required to be out on the hunt for perhaps a more beautiful mate but at a significant cost. However, had his house staffer been taking birth control pills, she likely would not have been secreting the engaging odors. As mentioned earlier, birth control pills mimic pregnancy and cause a type of pheromone to be released that indicates temporary infertility, signaling to males that she is not in the proper state for mating.

> When copulins are in the air, the male brain places less emphasis on factors like facial beauty, which is normally a very important indicator of health and vitality.

Keeping Him Close

In humans when a woman is ovulating it is more hidden than in other primates or species. Yes, the vagina does swell, but not very much, and usually, it is well hidden behind clothing most of the time. A woman however, does use exposed parts of her body to send a man subtle clues that she is ovulating, such as an ever-so-slight plumping of her lips, but these calling card clues are nowhere as overt as the external signs given by other primates.

Why humans have evolved to have sex for pleasure and not just for fertilization is debatable, but the prevailing theory is that a woman hides her fertility status in order to keep the man close. By having sex with him periodically, regardless of whether she's ovulating or not, she is more likely to keep him (and his important resources) nearby because he knows he has sex available to him. The most primitive part of the man's brain tells him this is good—he doesn't have to spend his resources or energy to go get another woman. In today's world, that means he doesn't have to spend money to court another female. I know this may sound awfully sexist, but females have motives as well as you will read ahead.

Women also detect pheromones, and nothing proves this better than the synchronized menstrual cycles of women living or working in close quarters. In one study, researchers found that just dabbing a bit of a woman's armpit secretions below another woman's nose allowing her to inhale the pheromones, would in turn alter her cycle (Preti, Cutler, Garcia, Huggins & Lawley, 1986). Many women have observed for themselves that menstrual cycles become synchronized in college dorms and offices where many women work and live together.

Evolutionary biologists believe the reason behind their synchronization is that women living together don't want to mate and have multiple offspring with the same male living in the household. In addition, most women living together are related and it wouldn't be genetically beneficial for a man to have sexual relations with partners who have similar genes. So, a woman's cycle will line up with those of all the women living under one roof, such as her sisters-in-law and housekeepers. Each female needs the household male to provide resources, so if multiple women were pregnant they would have to compete for resources. Theoretically, their synchronized systems create a small window of access to fertile cycles and the lord of the manor is most likely to only get one woman pregnant— unless, of course, he is "the Governator," Arnold Schwarzenegger.

Stronger Smellers

A common argument erupts as a young couple with a toddler debate whether or not a diaper change is needed for their young one. Both the father and the mother may be engaged in another activity that is garnering their attention however the mother seems more mindful to the necessity of their child. Is the father disengaged or does he just not realize the need for a diaper swap? As crucial as female pheromones are for signaling fertility status to men, women are the ones with a keener sense of smell. How do we know? One study revealed that women can pick out the odor of their own child, even if blindfolded, but males can't (Etcoff, 2000; Morris, 1997). And have you ever watched women shop for fruit and vegetables at a grocery store? Many of them pick up produce and sniff it, a behavior seen much more often in women than men. And although debatable, women also seem to smell a kid's dirty diaper long before her husband does.

> As crucial as female pheromones are for signaling fertility status to men, women are the ones with a keener sense of smell.

During ovulation, a woman's sense of smell is especially strong because it can help her stake out an ideal mate. (But again, birth control pills cancel this out because they mimic pregnancy. The body doesn't need this incredibly sensitive ability to smell male pheromones because she's not "on the market.") An ovulating woman will find the odor of symmetrical-looking, dominant males more pleasant, which is nature's way of highlighting their good genes. While this preference for symmetric men seems to affect both single and paired women, it is interesting that women who are already in a committed relationship tend to be even *more* attracted to a dominant male's odor.

Why the reasoning for a married woman to have a roving eyes and nose?

Mother Nature wants the best genes to win out, so even a woman with a man who is providing resources will, during her most fertile time, hunger after a genetically fit man who may be less invested in parenting, but carries strong, desirable genes she can transfer on to her offspring (Havlicek, Roberts & Flegr, 2005; Little, Jones, Penton-Voak, Burt & Perrett, 2002). In fact she is more likely to fantasize about a strong, strapping man with dominant features during ovulation.

> Mother Nature wants the best genes to win out, so even a woman with a man who is providing resources will, during her most fertile time, hunger after a genetically fit man who carries strong, desirable genes she can transfer on to her offspring.

Vive la Difference!

Another little-known fact about a woman's sex drive is that during ovulation, she will prefer and seek out a man who is least like herself—an MHC-dissimilar male. An MHC-similar man might be a blood relative, and partnering with him would go against the evolutionary goal of producing the best offspring possible. If we mate with someone close to our own genetic code, we increase the risk of genetic defects (Carrington et al., 1999; McClelland, Penn & Potts, 2003; Thursz, Thomas, Greenwood & Hill, 1997). Couples with similar genetic codes have longer intervals between children and more miscarriages (Ober, Hyslop, Elias, Weitkamp & Hauck, 1998; Ober et al., 1985). And similar genes between spouses may result in poorer relationships that are more likely to end in divorce (Voilrath & Milinski, 1995). This is the powerful natural basis that explains the reasoning behind social and religious bans on marrying close relatives—we create taboos and write laws to codify what we already know in human biology. Nature does not want us to pair up with someone who is genetically similar.

One study that confirms this fact as well as the role of scent in selecting a good match involved a hamper full of t-shirts that men had worn for several days. Women were asked to pick out the shirt they liked best, and that shirt would invariably contain an odor from an individual whose MHC-coded odor was most different from the woman's own. In addition, the shirt they liked *least* had an MHC-coded pheromone and odor most similar to their own (Wedekind & Füri, 1997; Wedekind, Seebeck, Bettens & Paepke, 1995).

> Nature does not want us to pair up with someone who is genetically close.

Nature covers her bases by adding a visual element to this distaste for similar genes, too. Women will judge the faces of men who are genetically similar to them as unattractive compared to men who have a very different genetic code (Roberts et al., 2005).

In spite of all the signals, sometimes MHC-similar couples do come together, of course, and when they do, nature doesn't cooperate very well. In a study of married couples with similar MHC, the women said that they were less sexually satisfied in the relationship, less likely to achieve orgasms, and more likely to have affairs. The men didn't report more affairs outside the relationship, but they did feel that their partners were less sexually satisfied. Overall, the more similar the partners' MHC, the less likely they were to be sexually satisfied (Garver-Apgar, Gangestad, Thornhill, Miller & Olp, 2006).

A woman has an incredible ability to recognize the scent of a biologically ideal mate, and if she is paired with someone who is not genetically ideal, she will subconsciously set up barriers to pregnancy, such as being uninterested in having sex and/or experiencing fewer orgasms, so that sperm has less chance of reaching an egg (Garver-Apgar, Gangestad, Thornhill, Miller & Olp, 2006).

When it comes to sniffing out a genetically ideal man, a woman's sense of smell is extremely fine-tuned. She'll be drawn to a man whose MHC is moderately different than her own, but *not* attracted to one whose code is vastly different. This way, nature tries to ensure that she won't have genetically weak offspring or get into a relationship in which the cultural divide would pose tough challenges for raising a child (Jacob, McClintock, Zelano & Ober, 2002).

We Just Can't Help It!

Performing surgery is an intensive exercise for both the mind and body. Most surgeons and operating room nurses work at a heightened state of attention with the same focus that drives a professional athlete during competition. Surgeons train for years, learning to block out distraction and center on the task at hand. That kind of intense focus raises adrenaline levels and, most likely, testosterone and pheromone output. After surgery, everyone throws their sweat- and pheromone-laced scrubs into a hamper, which is eventually hauled away by a laundry service.

Earlier in my practice I had a staff member whose job included managing the pickup and delivery of our scrub hamper. She was in her early thirties, single, and on a relentless search for her ideal match. One day, returning from surgery, I passed by her office and found her face buried in the scrub top of one of our male nurses, which she had obviously rifled out of overflowing hamper next to her desk.

She gave me a matter-of-fact look, shook her head, and said, "I just *love* this one's smell!"

It may be hard to accept that so much of our behavior—especially in the romance department—is dictated by underground processes we can't control. Nature has a prime directive that has been building a steam of momentum over millions of years and a few thousand years of civilization aren't going to stop it in its tracks. We can try to pretend it doesn't exist but better to understand and manage it than deny it.

Although most of us wear perfume, antiperspirants and deodorants to reduce body odor, these products may hurt our chances of finding Mr. or Ms. Right because they cover up our crucial MHC-coded pheromones. Without giving those molecules free reign, we hold back important genetic information that could attract the partner we've been waiting for. Maybe the French, who were late in adopting antiperspirants, were on to something.

The Real "Good" in Good and Plenty

That's not to say that perfumes and other nicely scented products are all bad. Odors do more than carry chemical messages about sexuality and fertility—there's evidence that certain smells, even in foods, can influence the impression you project to others. Alan Hirsch, one of the world's foremost experts in odor, has shown that smells can play games with our perception. Smelling pink grapefruit just before guessing a woman's age, for example, can result in her appearing up to five years younger than her actual age. For some reason that particular citrusy scent in your nose causes your brain to function differently! After researching with other foods like grapes and cucumbers, Dr. Hirsch discovered that

> Ruby Red Arousal: The scent of red grapefruit can increase blood flow to the penis up to twenty-five percent.

only grapefruit has this effect. His research also reveals that the smell of red grapefruit can increase blood flow to the penis up to twenty-five percent—an aroused state that could account for a man's sexual frame of mind that makes a woman appear youthful and sexually attractive.

Other smells known to increase penile blood flow include floral scents, and both cinnamon and lavender compel men to rate females more attractive, intelligent, successful, and trustworthy. So, next time you are in the mood or interested in gaining an advantage, there may be a benefit to bringing your partner breakfast in bed that includes a pink grapefruit, sprinkled with a little cinnamon and decorated with a flower.

Men, as well, may benefit from knowing what to bring their mate when they are feeling just right. Women as well respond sexually to scents, but the sources are quite a bit different. Hirsh learned that women are aroused by the combined smell of Good and Plenty candy, cucumber, banana nut bread, and pumpkin pie (Hirsch, 1998; Hirsch, Gruss, Bermele, Zagorski & Schroder, 1998). I am not sure if there is a recipe for a Good and Plenty/ banana bread sandwich which layered over a pumpkin pie but it may be worth a shot.

Kissing is more evidence of the link between smells and sexual excitation—when we kiss we benefit by getting our noses closer and smelling each other's unique scents. In fact, this may be the primary reason for kissing. And food has always been related to sex, which emphasizes how olfactory stimulation leads to sexual stimulation. In prehistoric times, the tribe would enjoy the meal following a hunt, and theoretically this would be the ideal time to procreate. Over the millennia and based on the success of this association, the scent of food odors came to increase genital blood flow and sexual attraction. As Dr. Hirsch remarks, "A relationship undoubtedly exists between the olfactory and sexual functions; its mechanism, however, remains to be discovered" (Hirsch 1999).

Most women realize the slimming effects of dark or vertically striped clothing or the way jewelry can draw attention away from another area. But many may not be aware that wearing a combination of floral and spice scents can make them appear up to seven percent thinner! In another study done by Dr. Hirsch, men wearing scarves sprayed with specific odors viewed a short, heavy female. When asked to estimate her weight, the men in scarves that carried the floral and spice combination estimated her weight at twelve pounds less than the men wearing scarves sprayed with other scents (Hirsch, Cohen & Carruthers, 2007).

> Wearing a combination of floral and spice scents can make a woman appear up to seven percent thinner!

Pleasant smells can change the way we perceive people and inanimate objects such as art, improve our mood, and stimulate our sexual juices. Bad smells, on the other hand, make us find people and things *less* attractive. It's no wonder, then, that the U.S. fragrance industry is expected to be worth $33 billion by 2015 (Global Industry Analysts, February 2011).

There is much more to scent than we think, and we're programmed to depend on this sense in order to find an ideal partner. Our personal scent is our calling card that introduces our background, health, and level of attractiveness to the world, and this fact makes a strong case against arranged marriages, in which someone else chooses our mate.

We know what is best for us and can smell it.

CHAPTER 6

ONE-NIGHTER OR
SOUL MATE?

Matchmaker Matchmaker,
Make me a match
Find me a find,
Catch me a catch
Matchmaker, Matchmaker...
For Papa, Make him a scholar
For Mama, Make him rich as a king
For me? well, I wouldn't holler
If he were as handsome as anything!

The award winning musical, *Fiddler on the Roof*, takes place in Tzarist Russia circa 1905. A peasant milkman, Tevye, the father of five daughters is intent on them marrying someone who follows in his traditions. The three eldest daughters wanting to please their mama and papa sing to the local matchmaker, Yenta, to find them the perfect match. The daughters each dream of meeting a handsome, smart and wealthy man, but also a catch who will meet with their parents' approval. But as this fateful story goes each of the three girls falls in love with the one who doesn't meet her parent's approval.

As I have shown, there are raw, biologically influencing forces that direct us to an ideal mate. On a subconscious level, we are stimulated by factors such as pheromones, dilated pupils and waist-to-hip ratio. We have little conscious control over these forces. For example, just as we are designed be repulsed at the notion of romantic involvement with a close relative, nature has designed us to desire a mate genetically very different from ourselves, ensuring the best possible combination of genes. But it may not be simple or efficient to find an exotic mate from a faraway land. And while there is a subconscious drive towards finding a mate who's genetically dissimilar, there is also the conscious pursuit of a potential mate without expending the energy, time or resources that may be required to find that person who is vastly different. Once we find the perfect mate, we are designed to procreate and produce genetically superior children. We are then given the responsibility to rear the offspring to an age at which they can be self-sufficient. As we age, our desires in a mate no longer center on procreation, but more on a partner with whom we can share a quality of life, gather resources for grandchildren and finally share the pleasures and challenges associated with our mature years.

Yenta and matchmakers

But there must be a reason why matchmakers have been around since the beginning of time. Arranged marriages are controversial and the infamous theme of many movies plays and books. From *Fiddler on the Roof* to *Pocahontas* they tap into our visceral core. To some, it is a crude primitive jail sentence, while for others a reassuring life buoy, helping to navigate rough waters of mate selection. While a third party person who knows your culture may be well-aware of what you desire in a home life, religion or culture, they may not be privy to what scents you crave or who may be your ideal genetic match. In cultures where arranged marriages are common-place, they may lead to adverse consequences for physical, mental and emotional well-being and constitute a barrier for continued education(Ertem & Kocturk, 2008). Moreover, arranged marriages may not be an efficient model of marriage, especially in the modern world where divorce is more tolerated (Dnes & Rowthorn, 2002). This is not to say that all arrangements are bad. In many cultures, young adults are arranged with a mate, ensuring commitment from both extended families toward the union's success.

> Arranged marriages could lead to a less adapted sect over generations—one that would be pushed to the fringes of existence.

Marriage is so much more than just mating. It is the cornerstone of society and without it there would be no civilization. In essence, marriage can be thought of as a human adaptive trait as well. Many arranged marriages are based on convenience or benefits for the well-being of the family or children. When two families decide to marry their children it may mean more combined resources for their offspring. Remember, grandparents are just as interested in the survival of their genetic material, which now happens to be living on in their grandchildren. They feel obligated to ensure their survival. And two individuals may get married against their biological wishes, but eventually grow, learn to live together and build a happy life within the context of their culture. However, this doesn't mean that they are the best combination. In fact, it is likely that there is someone out there better for them, a match with whom they would create more genetically fit children. Nevertheless, if that ideal mate is from too far "over the other side of the tracks" and doesn't fit into their strict culture then that genetically superior person may be forced out of the marriage and family. Ultimately this causes the children to suffer as they may be depleted of potential resources. Therefore, an arranged marriage in a strict culture loaded with restrictions may make sense. However, though, if the marriage partners are too closely related and isolated from other populations, theoretically it would eventually lead to a less adapted sect over generations- one that would be pushed to the fringes of existence.

Does speed dating make sense?

My cousin, the very good-looking former male model, that I have mentioned before is a serial dater. His first dates are always limited to a quick drink at a local bar. He tells me that he rarely takes his first dates to dinner because it only takes a few minutes to know if there is chemistry. He is not the only one to believe this. Studies show that within 30 seconds, we can accurately judge if we are interested in the opposite sex (Houser, Horan, & Furler, 2007). And if my cousin doesn't immediately feel sparks, he doesn't want to get dragged into a long dinner. In other words, he doesn't want to expend the resources (money) if he knows there is no potential for going further. Although I think my cousin could use a few lessons from Miss Manners, as a professor who does research in first impressions, this makes a lot of sense to me.

> It only takes us thirty seconds to accurately judge if we are interested in someone of the opposite sex.

When the concept of speed dating became popular in 1998, I was intrigued. Originating in Los Angeles, it quickly spread throughout the world. In speed dating, a group of single men and women congregate at a restaurant or large hall. Organized in a round-robin manner, they go from table to table meeting new members of the opposite sex. They spend five to eight minutes in conversation and then quickly rush off to the next table to meet another potential mate. At the end of the session, they put together a list of those they liked and the organizers facilitate a meeting between them. This concept intrigued me because such dating mechanisms validate the importance of first impressions. All it takes is 30 seconds, for most of us know fairly accurately if we are sexually attracted

However, in a modern world of baggy clothing, perfumes, colognes and birth control pills, many of the subconscious signals we send out are masked, hidden or abbreviated and therefore more difficult to pick up.

to another individual. So, why spend more time and resources than necessary? Speed dating allows an efficient and rapid scan of a group of individuals from the opposite sex to immediately determine who would make the best mate (Todd, Penke, Fasolo, & Lenton, 2007). To our prehistoric ancestors, this would have been ideal as we are designed to quickly evaluate, smell and identify the best mate for us. However in a modern world of baggy clothing, perfumes, colognes and birth control pills many of the subconscious signals we send out are masked, hidden or abbreviated and therefore more difficult to pick up. Speed dating would make more sense if we were to do it in loin cloths around a campfire. However, that may not be the most acceptable way to find our ideal mate in a modern world.

The evolution of on-line dating

"Hi I am in my early thirties, 6"2', dark-haired athletic, financially well off, a business owner earning more than 300K per year, professional, know what I like but always willing to listen to others' point of view. I enjoy travel, books and romantic adventures. And I am interested in meeting a woman who is sure of herself attractive in her demeanor and actions and ready for fun. Although previously shied away from long-term relationships now ready for something more meaningful with the right person."

"Hi I am a 28 year old 5"6' 105 lbs. long blonde hair, former competitive dancer now turned VP of creative agency. I enjoy what I do but not defined by it. Graduated from a large state school and received my Masters in literature from Princeton. Grew up in the suburbs but now live in city, enjoy boats, adventurous foods and reading the newspaper on Sunday Morning. I hunger for exotic activities in far -away lands and can't wait to plan my next trip. My favorite movies are in black and white and when in the end the guy always gets the girl. Although, I enjoy dancing till sunrise every once in a while, am just as pleased with a Saturday night on the couch sipping a glass of fine wine between handfuls of popcorn. I enjoy cooking and eating, and while not crazy about dishes hate a mess. I thrive on understanding what it takes to make others happy. Looking for a spark from a modern man who wants to have fun but willing to consider something more meaningful if the conditions are just right."

Wow! Both sound pretty good. What do you imagine they look like? Too good to be true? Are these would be lovers accurate in their descriptions?

The 21ˢᵗ Century, speed dating has been replaced by online dating services. According to *Online Dating Magazine* (http://www.onlinedatingmagazine.com/), about 5% of internet users have paid to use an online dating service (Jansen, December 30,

2010), 17% of couples that were married in the last three years met on an online dating service and one out of every five singles in the United States has dated someone they met online (C. M. Bailey, April 10, 2010). Online dating is the third most popular way for singles to meet, behind school/work and friend/family member. Money spent on online dating services and personal ads is predicted to dramatically increase. (Jupiter Research, February 2008).

So, why are online dating services so popular? It is likely because it allows us to scan even more individuals in a quicker period of time and spend even fewer resources (time, energy and money) than speed dating. A potential mate-seeker can view thousands of profiles in one evening. Hunting men can scan photos to identify who has the most symmetric facial appearances and shapely figures and discerning women can read biographies to identify the most resourceful dapper males. Some services won't suggest a potential male mate to a female if he earns less money than her. This is an evolutionary adaptive mechanism in a world in which physical clues are being further hidden.

Unfortunately, most online dating users don't tell the truth. In fact, one study shows that most men lie about their height and income- they really are two inches shorter and make 20% less than they admit.

Unfortunately, we tend to have inflated views of ourselves and when veiled behind the pixels of a cyber-screen many online daters don't tell the truth. In fact, one study shows that most men lie about their height and income- they really are two inches shorter and make 20% less than they admit- and females fib about their weight and age(McCarthy, 2009) But, assuming in a perfect world that the reported physical attributes were a true representation of actual physical appearance and status, why go out to the clubs or bars when you can comfortably and without risk, scan even more individuals in a quicker period of time? Eventually, however, you will still have to meet and see if the profile was accurate. Then, even more importantly, you can determine if there is "chemistry" between the two of you. I would suggest that this chemistry really refers to our individual scents or pheromones. I would propose that online dating services would be even more successful if there was a way to digitally capture our scents and electronically transmit them to potential mates even before meeting. How about a new dating company perhaps called: smell-harmony. com or smatch.com?

Are we meant to be monogamous?

Despite the fact that many men and women jest about the restrictions, studies have shown that married men live longer and healthier lives (Murray, 2000). However, some men, regardless of the health benefits to being married and especially if they possess highly symmetric features or abundant resources, will be driven by an evolutionary encoded urge to wander.

Remember, as humans, our biological goal on earth is to procreate and our bodies were designed to live to an age closer to 40- than 80. Polygamy wouldn't be adaptive or beneficial for our species in general unless the males had endless resources to support the many children. However every culture does have a few men in such a predicament, America has many wealthy rock stars, politicians and executives who are famous for fathering children with the "other" woman. And in cultures that have kings or supreme rulers with enormous wealth and power, it is not uncommon for him to have concubines and multiple children. In fact, the Sharifian Emperor of Morocco, Ismail the Bloodthirsty (1672-1727), is reputed to have had at least 888 children- although mathematically this seems rather impossible. However, from JFK to Bill Clinton to Silvio Berlusconi and Arnold Schwarzenegger, we see versions of modern day leaders with access to significant resources succumb to their primitive urges.

It's almost as if society expects this behavior from powerful men. From an evolutionary biologist's perspective, this can be explained as human nature. However, this wouldn't work for the majority of individuals in our society because a father would have to deliver resources to multiple children who would likely go hungry and not develop to the best of their abilities. Not to mention they likely would become emotionally affected as well, a father has more of an impact on his child's development then just being a breadwinner. But this doesn't change the fact that the male brain is prewired to find fertile females and drive for sexual intercourse. In fact, when questioned about the ideal number of sexual partners they desired in a lifetime, men mentioned 18, whereas women in the same survey indicated only four or five (Buss & Schmitt, 1993).

> In fact, when questioned about the ideal number of sexual partners they desired in a lifetime, men mentioned 18, whereas women in the same survey indicated only around 4 or 5.

Men and women are just as at odds when it comes to their views of random sex. If a man acts on his primitive urges and asks a woman he's just met to have sex with him, provided he doesn't get slapped, what are the chances she would say yes? How about the other way around, how many men would agree to have sex with a random female who offered? These very questions were tested in a study done on a college campus in Florida.

When men randomly approached women and asked them to have sex, zero percent of the women agreed. Then the situation was reversed, and women approached men and asked the same thing. Seventy-five percent of the men agreed to have sex! How different can men and women be? However, fifty percent of both sexes agreed to go on a date with a random stranger (Clark & Hatfield, 1989). The real take away from this study, as I see it, is that even total strangers have a fifty percent chance of getting a "yes" to the invitation for a date.

While polygamy for the masses doesn't make evolutionary sense, an eighty-year stretch of monogamy may not be ideal for the adaptive evolution of our species, either. It is more likely that the most genetically fit humans are designed for serial monogamy or a series of relationships in succession—at least until an age when they are no longer fertile or capable of supporting additional children.

> While polygamy for the masses doesn't make evolutionary sense, an eighty-year stretch of monogamy isn't ideal for the adaptive evolution of our species, either.

Why men and women are so different when it comes to sex

From a biological perspective, following pubescence, we are driven to procreate by urges beyond our comprehension that are dictated by the prehistoric, primitive part of our brain. Ultimately, we want to find the ideal mate and our senses are designed to seek them out. How is this done? We rapidly scan all the potential beings of the opposite gender to see if they may be a fit. Males are designed to be the initiators, and their brains are more likely to think a female is interested in him even if she isn't. This is adaptive because a male has to be excited in order to inseminate a female. In fact, men will widely pursue all who qualify once a certain threshold of attractiveness is met (Todd, et al., 2007). A female's risk is, however, high following sexual intercourse because she may be left pregnant and with a dependent child after nine months.

> It is adaptive for a female to be more choosey and much more selective.

It is adaptive for a female to be more choosey and much more selective. She wants to be certain she has found the right mate both in the immediate term for his sperm quality and in the long term for his resource providing capabilities. Does this better explain the behaviors we see at the local singles bar?

Ideally, males on the hunt for a mate would search for a female virgin because she obviously isn't pregnant or lactating and isn't burdened with other children to care for at home. Consider the following, hypothetically, a woman's reproductive life spans from ages 16 to 42, and for 99% of our evolution, there was no oral contraception pills. So if a female gets pregnant and delivers a baby early into her reproductive capable years and then is breast-feeding or getting pregnant continuously after her first baby, then she would only have 31 ovulatory cycles over her reproductive life or 1.18 per year. And if you recognize that during a menstrual cycle, there are only three days of fertility in which the egg is likely to be fertilized by the sperm, that would mean a female is only capable of conceiving in 93 of the 9,490 days of her reproductive life (Small, 2011). This is perhaps why men are adapted to go after younger women; he is biologically prewired to find the female that is most likely to get pregnant and, therefore, should dedicate his time and resources on a virgin. She would be the most ideal mate to result in fertilization and production of an offspring. This is why the male's subconscious mind searches for physical clues of virginity and why he likes clear, lighter-colored skin, a waist-to-hip ratio of 0.7, full breasts and buttocks. After having a baby, a female's skin often darkens, her breasts may drop from breast-feeding, and her hips and waist may become altered from the physical trauma and other changes that occur to the pelvis during childbirth. Although these changes may be mild or subtle, the human male brain is designed to identify these clues.

Females, on the other hand, are designed to identify the most resourceful males. In order to produce the most robust and viable offspring, they are seeking out the best provider and one dissimilar from their own genetic code. Females are prewired to be observant for any sign that a man is a holder of good genes. Her desires and abilities to identify those with good genes may be heightened during periods of fertility. And, as we have shown in Chapter three, ovulating women preferentially desire a more symmetric-appearing male. She also will desire a certain smell (S. W. Gangestad & Thornhill, 1998), facial evidence of masculinity (Johnston, et al., 2001; Penton-Voak, et al., 1999), social presence and dominance (S. W. Gangestad, et al., 2004) and a deeper voice (Puts, 2005). These are all signs that a male, in the short-term, will provide sperm with strong dominant genes. Ovulating women also are more likely to sneak out of their committed relationship and have an affair with a good gene provider. Furthermore, there is evidence that up to 10% of woman in some communities may have reached outside her relationship to become pregnant by someone other than her committed mate! (R. R. Baker & Bellis, 1995; Cerda-Flores, Barton, Marty-Gonzalez, Rivas, & Chakraborty, 1999).

However, when she is not ovulating, other traits may become more important or valued. A female may desire more feminine and less dominant traits in a male which she interprets as evidence he will be a loyal and good provider. Additional signs a female may look for include intelligence and creativity, both of which may indicate not only more access to material possessions and resources, but also traits that may be passed along to her offspring. And indeed, studies have found that both intelligence and creativity are important to a female's rating of attractiveness during and following ovulation (Prokosch, et al., 2009). As the relationship deepens and more interaction occurs, a mate's intelligence contributes a larger portion of what defines "mate appeal."

Does your level of beauty depend on who you hang out with?

A man on the prowl for a new mate would be better off taking his very attractive sister or female cousin with him to the bar. He is more likely to gain the interest of an attractive woman if he is with a beautiful woman then by being flanked with a group of ten meat head guys who look like pack of hungry hunters.

Females are searching for clues of health and wealth. In order not to waste as much time finding the perfect mate, a female becomes more interested if she sees a man with another attractive female. This is called "copying, "which means women tend to find other men with beautiful women more attractive because it indicates that the other woman did her homework. It is implied that she researched the mate and already determined he is a good genetic catch. But the key element here is the level of attractiveness of the woman who is accompanying him. If she is relatively unattractive then her value at increasing his stock is negligible but if she is gorgeous he looks like a rock star. And the research show that up to two-thirds of men said that they were successfully lured away by another woman (Buss & Schmitt, 1993). Interestingly, if a man wears a wedding ring, that by itself doesn't increase a female's level of attraction to him. (Little, Burriss, Jones, Debruine, & Caldwell, 2008).

> A female becomes more interested if she sees a man with another attractive female.

A beauty queen may be the belle of her local ball, but if standing next to Cindy Crawford she may look fairly average and she knows it.

Whom we are attracted to as a mate and our perceived attractiveness may be dependent on whom we stands next to and what season it is. This is based on the "contrast effect" theory. Most women know it but may not want to admit there is intense competition amongst young ladies to look good and outshine their neighbor. It is one of the reasons women are quick to criticize another's appearance. If they can outshine the women next to them, they may be more likely to get the male with the most resources. There is a biological reason for this because when people are exposed to an attractive stimulus, they will rate their own attractiveness and other surrounding stimuli as less attractive (Geiselman, Haight, & Kimata, 1984; Kenrick, Gutierres, & Goldberg, 1989; Kenrick, Montello, Gutierres, & Trost, 1993; Kowner & Ogawa, 1993). In a 1977 study conducted at Montana State University, this behavior was coined the "Farrah effect." Eighty-one undergraduate men were asked their opinion of photographs of potential blind-dates either before or after watching episodes of the infamous 1970s TV show "Charlie's Angels" staring three beautiful women lead by the 1970s sex symbol Farrah Fawcett. The men who were asked to rate the photo just following watching the show rated the females significantly lower than men who were not watching the show (Kenrick & Gutierres, 1980). Likewise, males exposed to pornographic films temporarily find their mates less attractive. However, it is time limited, as the male returns to his baseline existence. But the

> A beauty queen may be the belle of her local ball, but if standing next to Cindy Crawford she may look fairly average and she knows it.

male who happens to work or live in an environment full of beautiful women may have an extraordinary rating system of what he finds attractive. For the unattractive male, this can be particularly adverse as he develops unrealistic expectations and is never quite satisfied with the women who are available to him.

By this same contrast theory, a study done in Poland revealed that when in a cold season or environment where women are bundled up in clothing hiding all their physical assets, men become even more attracted to seeing body shapes and breasts than if in a warm environment and seeing it every day (Pawlowski & Sorokowski, 2008). So, for women living in a cold wintery climate wanting to look very attractive to men with resources, your best bet is to go to the luxury gym in town with an unattractive friend and wear a figure enhancing tight spandex outfit.

Infidelity

What if a male partner does cheat and commits an act of infidelity - how upset does his female mate become? Well, yes, pretty upset of course, but does it matter if the "other woman" is attractive? And how much does it matter if the excursion has no emotional involvement and was just a physical encounter? A study asked university campus students about their partner's infidelity and whether the attractiveness of the other partner mattered. The results show that regardless of attraction level, women were upset if her man strayed to another female- how attractive the other woman was didn't matter. It is just the fact he slept with someone else that bothered her. However, when asked if she would be more upset if he also committed an emotional infidelity, meaning he felt something for the other woman other than just a physical act, females were more upset if the other woman was attractive (Wade, 2006). This was confirmed in another study (Buss, Larsen, Westen, & Semmelroth, 1992), in which both men and women were asked to imagine their mate had an affair and then which bothered them more: the sexual or emotional infidelity? Well, what do you think? Among men, 61% judged the sexual infidelity the most upsetting compared to 13% of women. Conversely, only 39% of men, but 87% of the women judged the emotional attachment to the opposite sex more upsetting.

> Females were more upset if the other woman was attractive than if she was unattractive only if her partner was also committing emotional infidelity.

This would make sense because a female doesn't want her resource provider to divert his rewards to another mate and children. Deep down, she probably realizes that while a man may sleep around, it is much more of a threat if he is emotionally interested in an attractive woman because this would be a greater long-term threat to her resources.

We don't like to be poached of our mate. This is defined as behavior designed to lure someone who is already in a romantic relationship. According to one study, 60% of men and 53% of women report having attempted to poach or "steal" someone from an existing relationship (Buss & Schmitt, 1993). We will do our best to guard against this and despite the fact that poaching is widespread; we have developed tactics and emotions to stop it. When a female feels competition, she will put down her competition by denigrating the other woman's appearances; however, this is in contrast to men who, when jealous of losing their mate, will denigrate the resource capabilities of the other male, calling him lazy or lacking ambition and clear cut goals (Buss, 2004).

Do we settle if we don't get the alpha male or supermodel?

Once we choose a mate, do most of us find our mate attractive or do we just settle and say, "Yea, my spouse is okay looking. It was the best I could do." If I asked you how physically attractive your mate is on a scale of "1-10"what would you say? Likely, if you were being candid you said around"8."Most people pick a mate they find beautiful, even if others don't. We tend to be attracted to someone of the same attraction level as ourselves and many of us consider ourselves around an"8."Attractive people like other attractive people and unattractive people like other unattractive people. However, unattractive people don't realize their chosen

> We tend to be attracted to someone of the same attraction level as ourselves.

partners are unattractive. In other words, people don't settle for someone less attractive. We end up mating and pairing up with people who we find attractive, regardless of what others think. In fact, we most commonly rate our partner an"8" out of "10" regardless of whether they are actually a "5" or a"6" as judged by others. Our perception of others' attractiveness is based on how we see ourselves and whom we think we can get. Studies have shown that having similar levels of attractiveness within a couple is a factor in early relationship success. Studies have also shown that those couples that rate themselves similarly are more likely to be satisfied (Gaunt, 2006).

Additional evidence proves those who are highly attractive or have high self-esteem are more likely to want to pair up with other attractive individuals. Yes, that's right; who you find attractive is also based on your own self-esteem. If you view yourself positively and feel good about yourself you will believe you deserve a more attractive mate. What's interesting in studies that evaluate attractiveness and self-esteem find no correlation between levels of self-esteem and actual objective attractiveness! Therefore, your self-esteem may be high regardless of how attractive you would be rated on an objective scale. This is significant because when your self-esteem is high you feel attractive, regardless of whether you would objectively be considered attractive by others. In other words, a positive image of yourself is just as important to obtaining an attractive mate as being objectively highly attractive.

So, if you think you are beautiful, you will likely pursue and become matched with someone more objectively attractive than yourself.

So, if you think you are beautiful, you will likely pursue and become matched with someone objectively more attractive than yourself. For males, once they accumulate resources their self-esteem tends to rise and they believe they deserve a more beautiful mate. In fact, their scale of what they define as beauty becomes skewed to a more attractive person. When they had fewer resources, they were attracted to a less objectively beautiful female. It is likely that their subconscious brain restricted the range of potential mates to someone they thought they could get. Why would it be evolutionarily advantageous to waste resources (energy) on someone who is likely to reject them? Therefore, they found someone many would consider a "6," but to them seemed to be an "8." However, after they gained resources and self-esteem, they now wanted someone objectively more attractive. They believed that the best mate for them would be someone regarded as an "8" or "9." The person they previously desired is no longer considered attractive to them. The newly invigorated self-esteem ridden person now sees their previous "8" as a "6" like everyone else.

But this crude biological system is not by any means prejudiced to one sex. In fact, females are driven by the same forceful biological desires to mate with the ideal resource provider. If her mate doesn't provide resources or live up to the promise he made to deliver she may feel the urge to move on to another male. On the other hand, when a female obtains her own level of resource stability, she no longer feels the need to rely on the resources of a male. While a resourceful male is still important to her mating choice, she can and will place equal or more value on the physical attributes of a male that indicate an ideal genetic code. Being symmetrical, strong, youthful, tall, with a full head of hair will become increasingly important to her. Perhaps this could help explain the "cougar syndrome" where a resource (financially) stable, middle-aged woman desires the highly attractive bar tending younger man (Koyama, McGain, & Hill, 2004)- can anyone say Demi Moore and Ashton Kutcher? Remember, if we look at where we came from we can better understand the motivations and actions of others.

Are we meant to sleep together every night in the same bed?

If we look back at our primitive ancestors, it helps us to understand our behaviors and desires. Before there were grocery stores and butchers, our prehistoric male ancestors were responsible for being on the hunt for weeks at a time, capturing valuable resources (food) for their families. The males sent out by the community were likely very strong and healthy and would bond with their male comrades while out on the hunt. After long, successful missions, they would probably return to their village desiring sexual relations. However, keep in mind; these males were not used to sleeping with their wives every night. They were in the wilderness with male co-hunters, working to bring home resources. Their female partner, who remained home, was taking care of the offspring, providing for them with whatever could be gathered easily, perhaps berries and grains. Lactating mothers would continue to feed their offspring for as long as they could with their own milk. This may go on until the child was six or seven years old. While producing milk for their young offspring, they would be releasing pheromones that would indicate to others they were not fertile.

> How many stories have we heard— whether true or not— about the male at work all day and his sexually deprived wife at home who eyes the attractive pool boy or trainer!

As a lactating female is not fertile, her internal biological forces also make her less interested in sex. Theoretically, any males left behind to protect the village would not be receiving any subconscious mating calls from these females to even pique their sexual interest. However, these males were also unlikely to be the most genetically fit. They probably were young, infirm or not very resourceful or strong. The strong males were out on the hunt. But once the female was done lactating and her offspring were of an age to provide for themselves, she now would become interested in becoming pregnant again and she would desire the most resourceful, genetically fit male around - especially if her partner or husband is gone on the hunt. How many stories have we heard - whether true or not - about the neglectful husband at work all day and his sexually deprived wife at home who eyes the attractive pool boy!

Although we have evolved and continue to do so, you can now understand where this behavior stems from. Interestingly, a male with ample resources may be interested in impregnating another female so long as he can afford to support another child. Mother Nature does not care if we have multiple partners as long as we can provide the necessary resources to enable that child to reach reproductive age. The critical responsibility for both parents is to get that offspring to a self-sufficient age so the child has the best chance to reach its genetic potential. Once again, we see how modern society and religion have interpreted and codified our biological urges by bestowing laws upon us, such as marriage contracts that place a requisite financial penalty on the male who leaves in order to ensure that children receive the necessary resources. Because without it, the children may be handicapped and disadvantaged before reaching the appropriate reproductive age, thereby not reaching their genetic potential. On a large scale, such behavior and consequences will hinder our species evolutionary adaption. Whereas during our ancestry, it was critical that the male provided resources for the first six or seven years of a child's life; today it is codified in law as 18 years of age.

How much have we changed over the thousands of years of evolution? Mate pairing for two individuals involves an implicit contract. In an evolutionary sense, and to our prehistoric ancestors during our period of greatest fertility, the man would agree to provide resources and the female agrees to stay attractive to her male. When one of them fails, the desire to search outside the relationship becomes greater.

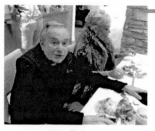

Uncle Jerry

Uncle Jerry always got his steak first.

After running the books for their business, preparing the house to host an extended family of 75, putting on a dress and looking attractive, my Aunt Marcelle would then serve dinner. But before any of the kids could eat, she made sure her husband, my Uncle Jerry, got served his steak first. The kids sat at the table and waited till Uncle Jerry was sitting down with his steak in front of him. This behavior was denigrated by my liberated American aunts and by the guest who would come to her house. Us progressive kids who grew up in American culture thought it was awfully primitive and backwards, especially growing up in the enlightened 70's. But Aunt Marcelle wasn't the only one who both worked in an office by day and practiced treating her husband like a king in the evening. All five of my aunts who were very traditional and Moroccan in some ways but very modern in other areas did the same. But perhaps they knew something important to our evolutionary make up. In our social contract that Mother Nature asks us to commit to when we pair off: a wife is responsible to make their husbands feel special and to stay attractive to him. The husbands in return are responsible to always provide resources, while protecting and treating her like a queen. When one party fails to uphold their end of the agreement then the relationship may suffer. Today we have marriage contracts and religious guidelines to keep us committed, but to humans monogamous relationships are beneficial to the individuals and the children for as long as both continue to keep up their end of the deal.

> Human adaption has not yet caught up with our advancing society.

Legally enforced and mandated inequality of rights has proven to lead to destruction of societies, however, the expectations of equal rights as related to behavior that go to the opposite extreme and don't recognize differences in the genders may negatively impact society as well. While we like the idea of comprehensive equal rights, Mother Nature has yet to make the genders behave identically. We don't have all the same urges, desires and needs. So while social and political equal rights are important and critically necessary to a society's existence, being sensitive to gender may make sense when judging the parameters of equal rights within a familial unit. Maybe we miss the mark when we demand women to dress in men's clothing, or when we expect men, in order to prove their humanity, to be expressively sensitive. While behavioral equal rights sounds politically like a good idea in its modern form it may actually go against some of our natural pre-wired urges. Equal rights, as discussed in the contemporary westernized world, may suffer if making those whose practices are different and biologically rooted seem bad and/ or wrong. Looking back now, I think my aunts were on to something. Yes, they are special and they felt every bit equal in the relationship and because they cooked or were the primary caretaker of the young children they didn't feel denigrated. They felt empowered and were proud to fulfill such roles. These roles were celebrated in their culture and upbringing. Conflict in society, politics and law often occurs when we try to mandate going against our natural urges. Yes, measures to discipline ourselves against destructive natural urges in a modern society are necessary to a successful civilization. But if we are going to best control them, it is also important to realize why these urges occur. Once we do they seem easier to conquer and deal with both on a personal level and on a societal level. And human adaption has not yet caught up with our advancing society. Look no further than sugar. As I sit here eating my fourth cookie, I realize that our primitive urges still want and desire sugar and when it's readily available it's hard to avoid eating it. But until our bodies adapt and develop the

> Equal right as discussed in the contemporary westernized world may suffer if making those whose practices are different and biologically rooted seem bad and/or wrong.

gene to turn off our insatiable desire for sugar, obesity and diabetes will continue to plague our modern societies.

How important is pillow talk after sex?

Are you surprised to learn that men will exaggerate the depth of their feelings to gain sexual access (Haselton & Buss, 2001)? In other words they may be over the top with the flattery just prior to getting a woman into bed, but unfortunately, their feelings change after they achieve orgasm. Men experience decreased sexual attraction to their partner immediately following sexual intercourse (Haselton, Buss, Oubaid, & Angleitner, 2005). Social scientists call the period of time after sex until one falls asleep or leave the "post coital time interval" (PCTI).

> Paradoxically, the less males talked about their commitment to the relationship, the more they were satisfied with this time period and their female partner!

Wouldn't you know it - this time period is more important to females than males, especially those females who are interested in long-term relationships. A study of 160 college students surveyed the importance and satisfaction of the PCTI. For females interested in more long-term commitment, they wanted to talk and discuss relationship bonds, trying to further the commitment of her male; however, if she was not interested in a long-term bond, she found this time less important. Paradoxically, the less males talked about their commitment to the relationship, the more they were satisfied with this time period and their female partner! So, it is ironic that a female wanting to keep a man close might be better off not discussing her desire to bring him home for the weekend to meet her mother immediately after having sex (Kruger & Hughes, 2010).

'Til death do us part

Today, most of us make religious vows during marriage ceremonies. However, 200,000 years ago, when two humans decided to form a monogamous union with intent to procreate, they had to comply to an implicit contract that was yet to be codified in written law. A give and take, or yin and yang as the Chinese say, has always been part of the natural law and it still exists today. As mentioned previously, the male implicitly promises he will provide resources for the female and their offspring until the child reaches a self-sufficient age. If he cannot uphold his end of the bargain, she has the right to leave to find a better male suitor. Does this sound crude and uncivilized? Well, yes perhaps, and keep in mind there are many exceptions, but would it surprise you that one of the main reasons for divorce in

> It does make evolutionary sense that when the male cannot provide for the female, she may lose attraction to him.

modern society is financial hardship (Bloom, Niles, & Tatcher, 1995; Burkett, 1989; Lown & Chandler, 1993; Poduska & Allred, 1990)? Although the data is debatable, it is widely perceived as a major cause for divorce. It does make evolutionary sense that when the male cannot provide for the female, she may lose attraction to him, and while she doesn't want to admit it consciously, perhaps it is a subconsciously influenced decision. On the other hand, a male who has achieved the necessary level of resourcefulness will expect his female to care for their children and remain physically attractive to him or else he will feel the right to leave for a more ideal mate. Does that sound horrible as well? It certainly does, but the social sciences show that males with higher self-esteem and resourcefulness believe they are deserving of a more attractive mate. Furthermore, resourceful males often want a more attractive female. So, what does this cold data mean to us today and how can we interpret it? For the male wanting to keep his beautiful wife and kids close, he will feel pressure to provide continuous resources or risk losing his mate. For the female, it means physically maintaining herself and providing an attractive image to her spouse. Yet, modern society is quickly adapting and evolving toward a new order.

Today, a female who is financially independent and has the ability to garner her own resources no longer feels dependent on the male partner, and if she doesn't desire him or need him sexually anymore, she is more likely to stray. In fact, females who rate themselves as more feminist are less concerned with the financial success of their male (Koyama, et al., 2004). This may be one of the reasons females who achieve financial independence are more likely to get divorced (Ermisch, 1993). As there are many more females now that are financially independent, males today may be feeling less pressure to achieve and provide continuous resources. Therefore, we are evolving toward a more egalitarian relationship between the genders, but keep in mind that evolution works over eons- not decades. So, while our laws and social mores of today attempt to follow a righteous and politically correct path, our brains and our DNA are still encumbered with the forces of natural selection that have been shepherding us for over four million years.

Endless Love and Marriage

Early on in my career I saw in consultation a retired sports announcer who liked to talk about the ponies. A salty fellow with a squint and crooked smile, he had no interest in cosmetic treatments, but he was referred to me for removal of a skin cancer from his forehead. After my treatment, the cancer was cured, he did well and years later I saw him back because he developed a twitching disorder around his eyes, a neurological condition that is treated with Botox. I started treating him periodically and we got to be friendly and talked a lot. He felt comfortable telling me that he never got married and I asked him why and he said that he was sorry he missed out on the love of his life who married someone else. Years later on a Valentine's Day he comes in with a woman who he had recently met. She was a very nice, attractive and well put together, mature lady in her late 70's and she was interested in treatment for wrinkles.

I had the opportunity to talk with the two of them and they began to tell me their story. They recently were reacquainted at their 50th year high school reunion. She was married twice with six grandchildren and her latest husband recently passed away. But when Frank said to me in his gruffy voice, "Doc, remember the love of my life I told you about a few years back?" "Yes of course." I said. "Well here she is and she looks no different than she did when she was 18!" For Frank she was the high school sweet heart he loved and waited 50 years to get. And he couldn't be more thrilled. I learned a few lessons here. One is sometimes it takes a long time before you finally meet your sweet heart and secondly once you find the love off your life he/she never changes. They got married, which doesn't make sense from an evolutionary standpoint as it would seem biologically unnecessary; however, there are benefits to marriage beyond procreation.*

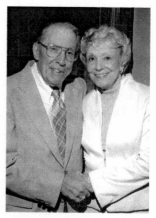

Frank and his lovely wife

The Benefits of Marriage

> But the marriage has to be right; if marriage is of a poor quality the benefits from remaining married are no longer and it is actually a detriment to health and economic well-being.

The comfortable feelings of marriage, union and sharing go beyond a drive to spread your seed. Although much more significant for men, both married men and women live longer and healthier lives (Waite 2003). Marriage is associated with greater overall happiness and married men earn more money than their never married counterparts. But the marriage has to be right, if marriage is of a poor quality the benefits from remaining married are no longer and it's actually a detriment to health and economic well-being. Unhappily married people experience increased adverse immunological effects and increased risk of illness. Being married means having someone who can provide emotional support on a regular basis thereby decreasing depression anxiety and other psychological problems and improving overall mental health. It is important that we match up with the right mate even if we have to wait for him/her! If we follow our biological encoded natural urges when it comes to mate selection rather than committing to what others tell us is best we will be more apt to find our ideal mate. Listen to your gut.

The importance in making your spouse your friend

Every summer morning before day camp, when I was a preteen, I used to accompany my grandfather to his breakfast location. His routine was to meet with two tables of other men and they would sit, eat and debate the day's events. All of them retired with plenty of time on their hands, some of them were financially well off, others were not, but it seemed to matter very little. After breakfast, they would team up and go to the race track, run errands or hang out at the ballpark. From a 10 year old's perspective they seemed very content with their positions and stages in life. I would sit, listen and try to understand their discussions but of course it was above my head. However, I was perceptive enough to realize they all greatly enjoyed each other's company. Otherwise why return the next day?

Friends provide a source of comfort and well-being that we may not get from our families or spouses. Both men and women gain feelings of well-being and morale from friends, but women, the more socially investing gender benefit greater. Even more interesting, neither's interaction with family members has any appreciable effect on morale or emotional well-being! This sounds erroneous, but is true. The reason being, we choose our friends and they choose us, whereas children, while perhaps unconditionally loved, may present us with feelings of worry, obligation and concern. Our parents, while appreciated and honored, may require extensive care and attention. Friends on the other hand give and take from us more equitably and if not we can choose to unfriend them (Lee 1987). This phenomenon is consistent with the "Thrifty theory"; the less you take from a relationship, the longer it will last. Most any relationship, if you take fewer resources prolongs. This theory applies to the economy or the ecosystems, take less from the economy and money lasts longer, take less from the environment and it will last longer (Medical Hypotheses (2006) 67, 15–20). Those who take fewer resources from Mother Nature also live longer, the only proven way to extend life is to calorie restrict or eat less than is needed. And to take this one step further, take fewer resources from your spouse and your relationship may endure. In other words, give as much if not more than you get and longevity is the byproduct of the relationship. Obviously to some limit. Any rule can be followed too far and have the opposite effect. Give too much and be abused is the reversal. But if in moderation this theory proves very reliable. If we want family relationships to be less obligatory and more rewarding then there has to be equality in the give and take. Share your spouse's victories as well as nurture their wounds. Do less talking and more listening and the relationship will remain forever fruitful. The take from the story, to assure a happy marriage we should strive to be partners, lovers and most importantly, open minded dependable friends. (Research on aging vol 9, no 4. Dec 1987. 459 482. Lee GR Social interaction, loneliness and emotional well-being among the elderly study done on people over age of 55 in state of Washington in 1980 over 2700 participants)

> In other words, give as much if not more than you get and longevity is the byproduct of the relationship.

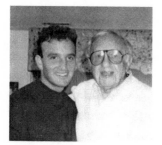

Me and my Grandfather
during my formidable years

Grandparenting

Grandparents are by nature invested into their grandchildren's health and well-being, because it is Mother Nature's designed pathway to genetic immortality. Within grandchildren resides a portion of the grandparents' DNA. And in many cultures the grandparents' involvement is integral to the raising of their grandchildren. These genetic guardians likely assume a responsibility to stay healthy and nurture their grandchild(ren) until they reach an age of self-sufficiency. My parents were divorced and I lived with my maternal grandparents growing up. My grandfather was not well but he assumed a burden having to take care of me and my sister. Nevertheless he survived until just after I graduated from medical school. I always felt that he somehow felt or knew that once I got through medical school his job was done. Supported by research that reveals women who have children at an older age live longer, being involved or committed to a process such as child rearing seems to prolong our lives (Rudi G. Nature, December 1998).

> Share your spouse's victories as well as nurture their wounds of defeat.

Look no further than the evolutionary reason behind menopause to see the evidence that grandparents or at least grandmothers are essential to the health and well-being of grandchildren. Humans living in the harsh environments of the primitive world needed to constantly adapt to survive and within that context menopause has evolved to help assure the grandchildren thrive. In multiple species the females and/or males soon die after reproducing, worst off is the Australian Redback spider who has sex once then immediately meets his demise, being eaten by his mate. But for humans, menopause has an evolutionary benefit because once a woman is past her reproductive years she can divert her attention to the care of her grandchildren. Unlike many species humans are born highly dependent on their mothers for survival. As a consequence of a large brain, fetuses are born earlier while their head and brain is still immature and small enough to fit through the birth canal, after which the brain finishes developing. But this delays independence and means a lot of energy must be spent by a mother helping to feed and care for young children until they develop to a stage of self-sufficiency. And if a mother has multiple children in short span it would be very difficult for her to fend for them all equally. However, a menopausal grandmother doesn't need to spend energy on her own children anymore; rather she can devote time to helping raise the next generation.

Alex's story

Soon after my middle child was born she developed a horrible gastrointestinal disorder. Her own immune system would attack and strangle the blood vessels to her small intestines periodically and randomly shutting down her entire digestive system. She would scream in pain and was unable to eat. It relegated us to many worrisome, sleepless nights in the hospital with her giving nutrients through her veins. Unfortunately, the physicians we sought weren't quite sure of why it was occurring. It didn't follow any normal or known disease patterns. There were many guesses but nobody was correct. We had no answers making it even more difficult. We didn't know if she was going to live or die. Between

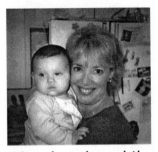

My mother-in-law and Alex

the uncertainty and watching her suffer in pain, in every way it was the worst time of my life. She was prescribed high dose steroids (and anti-inflammatory medication) as this seemed to work best to blunt the attacks. But the steroids had major side effects including stunting her growth. She remained on these and other powerful drugs during critical development stages leading to her adopting a funny appearance which attracted many curious stares. At the age of four she was barely two feet tall but could speak in full sentences. Others who didn't know of her arresting physical condition were so impressed by such a small young child that could talk so well. As parents though we were blinded to her physical impairments and thought she was the cutest thing in the world.

During her first five years of life, she would be in and out of the hospital and with two other needy young children at home my wife and I needed help beyond what a baby sitter would be expected to do. During this critical time in our daughter's life both grandmothers were

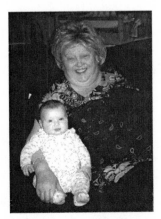

My mother and Alex

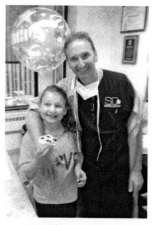

Alex and me

critical to our existence and Alex's well-being.

My Mother and Mother-in-law were always available, ready and willing to take on as much responsibility as necessary till we nurtured our daughter to health. Their help was absolutely essential and I don't know what would have transpired had it not been for their heroic efforts. It was clear to me that Mother Nature has made a natural role for grandmothers to want to help their grandchildren survive. Fortunately, when Alexandra reached the age of five the disease left as mysteriously as it had arrived, still no explanation for why or what was the cause. And I am happy to tell you that today Alexandra, is a thriving 11 year old who is the star of her soccer and basketball teams and has more compassion than any kid I know. She dreams of someday being a teacher for kids with special needs.

As we enter the mature stages of life, we feel an obligation to care and witness the success of our grandchildren. Our interests are less focused on mating and more on protecting resources for our children. However, we gain our strongest feelings of well-being from friends with whom we surround ourselves. At this stage in our lives, we seem to place greater emphasis on mates that make us feel better about ourselves. Men become less concerned about female body shape (Currie & Little, 2009) and more interested in other non-physical clues of attraction. And while strong evidence exists that sexual relations are still very important to mental well-being, many long-term relationships are driven more by the resource-sharing and emotional benefits gained from the relationship than the physical attributes previously emphasized (Levenson, Carstensen, & Gottman, 1993). Most studies show that as we age, satisfaction with our appearance, our lives and also whom we have chosen as partners tends to increase. As we age, we become smarter, and more accepting, of who we are and the choices we have made.

The Good Life Beyond Youth and Beauty

Just last year my grandmother passed away at the age of ninety-seven, or at least we think that was her age. We were never quite sure when she was born, but we knew she hailed from Casablanca, Morocco, where at age sixteen she met and married my grandfather, a dapper twenty-four-year-old banker from Marrakesh, Morocco. They moved to my grandfather's city and over the next sixteen years had nine children.

They lived in a close knit community with a strong tribal tradition in which all members of the community were regarded as family. Not until they were in their fifties did my grandparents move with the whole clan to Chicago and integrate into a culture that emphasized self-reliance and the individual more than the community. But they never abandoned their traditions, and in some respects clung to them with even greater intensity.

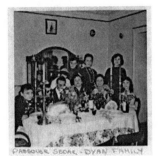

My Dad, his parents and sibling's family picture in Morocco

My aunts and uncles all married and raised their kids in the U.S., and my twenty-eight cousins and I saw each other all the time. We remained a close extended family, unlike the small nuclear family that had become the American standard. This was never clearer than when I graduated from medical school—while most of my fellow classmates walked across the stage to polite applause from their immediate families, I was greeted by the traditional shirking and tongue-rolling calls from a bursting crowd of "Rockin' Moroccans" standing in the back of the room.

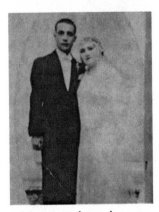

My paternal grandparents on their wedding day

But like so many other first- and second-generation Americans, my cousins and I slowly shed some of the practices of the old world. One tradition we haven't abandoned, however, is respect and reverence for elders in the family.

My grandfather passed away at age seventy-two, and as my grandmother went on to live another twenty-five years, family always surrounded her. She was never alone and always closely cared for. As she aged, her children and grandchildren never considered her a burden, but rather the family matriarch who evoked deep respect and love. As she neared the end of her life, my generation and the next would kneel at her bedside to receive her blessings, which we believed to be powerful and divinely inspired.

Like my Moroccan heritage, many cultures associate aging with wisdom and honor and consider the elderly worthy of the utmost respect. In the Asian cultures rooted in Buddhist, Confucian and Taoist philosophy, elders are a central part of the family and revered for their

> As we age, we become more psychologically resilient and are able to see the positives within negative situations more easily.

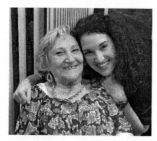

My sister and my paternal Grandmother in her 90's

knowledge and giving of wisdom. Elders are perceived as holding transcendental understanding and are a socially valuable part of life.

In contrast, American society tends to focus on the individual and how much we can accomplish and produce—as a result, when we retire and grow beyond our "productive" years, we can lose a sense of purpose and self-esteem. Yet, even with an overall lack of value placed on the mature generation, studies show that as we age we tend to be more accepting of who we are and our position in life.

We've learned that regardless of culture, older adults fare more favorably than younger adults when it comes to many different aspects of well-being (Karasawa et al., 2011; Collins and Smyer, 2005). As we age, we become more psychologically resilient and are able to see the positives within negative situations more easily. In other words, we're better at finding the silver lining.

> Older women are more satisfied with their bodies than younger women.

In a society like ours, where our ability to contribute to our social status and economic status is greatest during our young adulthood, self-esteem seems to rise until about age sixty and is related to our ability to be extraverted, optimistic and have control over our personal destiny. Even past the age of retirement, our optimistic ability to master our own destiny and be extraverted are buffers against a significant loss of self-esteem. Women seem to be especially empowered with aging, whether they live in a collective or more individual-oriented community. They find it liberating to no longer have the constant pressure of being defined by physical beauty. It might be logical to think that women would feel less happy with their bodies as they deal with the physical changes of aging, but in fact, older women are **more satisfied** with their bodies than younger women. Women seem to cherish older age and feel empowered by the self-esteem and confidence they gain (McMullin&Cairney, 2004). Higher self-esteem leads to happiness. And older women, who are more social than men, tend to have more friends, which also leads to greater happiness.

As we age, happiness and self-esteem are integrally related, yet different. In communities and groups where the collective is more valued than the individual, self-esteem is even less critical as a source of happiness (Lyumbomirsky, Tkach&Dimatteo, 2006). While self-esteem may decline in age for some who lose control of their destiny, happiness can still be robust regardless of a hopeless situation or negative circumstances such as employment, financial loss and poor health. Older people tend to manage loss better, relinquish unobtainable goals, and are accepting of who they are and what they have achieved. Happiness is more related to a positive mood, satisfaction with life right now, and social relationships with friends. Contentment with friendships is one of the biggest predictors of well-being at all ages, and older people have been found to report higher levels of happiness than younger ones (Roberts & Chapman, 2000; Sheldon & Kasser, 2001).

> Contentment with friendships is one of the biggest predictors of well-being at all ages.

Confucius wrote, "Old age, believe me, is a good and pleasant thing. It is true you are gently shouldered off the stage, but then you are given such a comfortable front stall as spectator." Our golden years can truly be the best time of our lives. Relieved of many of the competitive burdens and responsibilities of youth and middle adulthood, more willing to accept our station in life, better equipped to handle negative situations and buoyed by the enlightened feeling of accumulated experiences are the human formula for happiness in our mature years. And when we have the opportunity to pass wisdom on to an accepting younger generation, this stage of life can be even more gratifying, making our last decades the best of all.

CHAPTER 7

JUNK IN THE TRUNK

"Evolution is a tightly coupled dance, with life and the material environment as partners."

—James Lovelock

L ate last year I met a young man from Nigeria who came in for a consultation. He had moved to the United States and was making a life for himself in Chicago. Recently married and starting to plan a family, he wanted to undergo a nasal reshaping procedure to make his nose smaller. I was curious why he insisted on having it done so soon and prior to attempting to get his wife pregnant. Upon further discussion, I came to understand his motive for undergoing rhinoplasty. He was concerned that his children would have a wide nose like his, which he thought would make it difficult for them to blend in with friends and others in the community. To assure they didn't get his nose, he wanted to surgically reduce its size before they were conceived.

He had not been taught the concept of genetic inheritance, and I had to advise him that even if he did undergo a nasal surgery, his children would still inherit the genetic traits for the noses that have been in his family lineage for over hundreds of thousands of years. But the good news was that because he was marrying a Caucasian woman with a narrower nose, his children would likely have noses that were a blend of the two of them.

Why do populations from far corners of the earth look so different? People of sub-Saharan African descent are tall with dark skin and wide noses, while those of Eskimo ancestry tend to be shorter and heavier with thick brows and heavy eyelids. Like so many themes throughout this book, the answer lies in evolutionary adaption.

For people living near the equator, darker skin protects from the intense sun exposure, and if they are on the hot, flat African plains, being taller allows them to release body heat more efficiently and see further above obstructing brushes to spot potential game. In this humid environment, a wide nose allows people to quickly take in a lot of moist oxygen-air, in contrast to the cold, dry north, where a long, narrow nose is advantageous because it contains additional space to humidify and warm the air. For those living in the frozen tundra near the North Pole, a shorter, fatter body would have less surface area exposed to the cold and could conserve heat more efficiently. Additionally, heavy eyelids would protect from the chilly weather, wind and snow. It makes evolutionary sense that local populations over thousands of years would adapt to their environments and develop these physical traits.

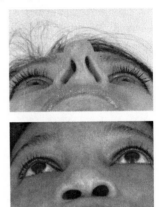

Different nostril sizes in different cultures are an evolutionary adaptive trait.

The Evolution of Miss Universe

The Miss Universe pageant was launched in 1952 by a California swimsuit company and has grown into a multi-million dollar venture, with women participating from all around the world. Its intended purpose, as reported in their creed, reads: "We, the young women of the universe, believe people everywhere are seeking peace, tolerance and mutual understanding. We pledge to spread this message in every way we can wherever we go."

In the pageant's early years, the most successful country was the United States, but in the past forty-two years there have only been three winners from the U.S. The choice of winners migrated toward the Latin Americas, in particular Venezuela and Puerto Rico, which became the most successful in the eighties and nineties with ten winners over a thirty-one-year span.

Today, the east, specifically India, is becoming a rising powerhouse in the pageant. The first black winner was from Haiti in

1992 and the first African crowned was Miss Botswana in 1999. And last year's winner, which included voting from the televised audience, was from Angola.

It's not uncommon for all the populated continents of the world to now be represented in the semifinals. What started out as an ethnocentric marketing investment for a swimsuit maker has now spread to a worldwide event in which women are judged attractive based on more than how they just appear in their swimsuits. The winner is also expected to be intelligent, well mannered, and cultured.

While the pageant may seem crude and shallow to some, in many respects it follows human evolution. For millions of years the female gender has been judged based on her physical assets that represent youthfulness, fertility, and femininity—however, much more goes into being attractive than just appearance, and the pageant seems to recognize this, at least on the surface. While each participant has won local and national competitions to be deemed the best of her country, as TV, movies and the Internet continue to shrink the world, our understanding and comfort level with what other cultures find attractive is becoming ingrained into our psyches. At the same time that we are becoming accustomed to seeing and recognizing what is beautiful from each culture, the winner of Miss Universe continues to evolve toward a blend of the best the multicultural world has to offer in both appearance and intelligence.

Although we all look slightly different based on our genetic lineage, do certain physical traits transcend geography and become cross-culturally consistent? In other words, would you perceive certain people from Ghana attractive if their own community of peers considered them attractive? While this may be difficult to process and we often limit ourselves to a specific "type" we find good-looking, the answer is yes. But it doesn't happen at first glance. There is usually an adjustment period before we're able to look beyond obvious differences in culture.

> Certain attractive facial characteristics associated with youthfulness are common across both Eastern and Western cultures.

When we first meet someone from a foreign culture, we tend to fixate on how different they look and find it nearly impossible to look past that. This is one of the reasons why a jury of our own peers is so critical in our legal system—eyewitnesses are less likely to misidentify someone from their own race (Wells & Olson, 2001).

Unfortunately, this difference is intimidating at first and has fueled some of humanity's greatest atrocities, from racism to genocide. However, after becoming accustomed to cultural and racial differences, we adapt and start to gain comfort and familiarity within the foreign culture. Eventually, we even adopt some of their cultural physical differences to our own internal references of beauty. Our local range of what we find beautiful changes, deviating in a direction of the average of all the people in the new population. Soon, we are able to assess the same people as attractive in the foreign culture that are considered attractive within their own community.

Nevertheless, certain attractive facial characteristics associated with youthfulness are common across both Eastern and Western cultures. Large eyes, petite chins, and translucent, homogenous, light-colored skin are always considered attractive. In Japanese culture, Geishas represent the height of beauty and servitude for men and are famous for their white faces. The heavy white paint, while not necessarily attractive to Westernized males, symbolizes what all humans identify as beautiful: a lighter complexion, which we equate with youthfulness. Likewise, sixteenth-century Queen Elizabeth I of England, who never married and was fixated on remaining youthful, is forever known as the Virgin Queen, clearly a term associated with youth, vitality, and promise. It is not surprising that this woman, who was likely well aware of human nature's fascination with youthfulness, became famous for her white, lead-painted face.

Although we find particular attributes attractive in females regardless of culture, humans can't help becoming fixated on their different facial structures and features when meeting another culture for the first time. In the words of standup comedian Dave Chappelle:

"If you call a Korean guy Chinese—I've done this—they'll flip out. 'Hey! What makes you think I'm Chinese? I am Korean! Do I look Chinese?'

"Yes, Man, you do look Chinese, that's why I said it. It was an accident. To an untrained eye you all look Chinese to me."

He's got a point: it takes a while to start to recognize and appreciate the slight differences in features of people of other cultures. After spending time in Asia, a naïve Caucasian will soon start to appreciate the subtle distinctions that are common to Korean, Japanese or Chinese appearances. After becoming familiar with the culture, he or she will begin to recognize the individuals that are considered beautiful in that society. As our modern civilizations become more multicultural, our frames of reference expand and ideals of beauty shift toward the average of the multiracial society. Therefore, people of a multicultural society tend to find someone who is a combination of the representative features of all the cultures as

> As our modern civilizations become more multicultural, our frames of reference expand and ideals of beauty shift toward the average of the multiracial society.

the most beautiful. Of course, this would make evolutionary sense because a person who has a multiracial, multicultural background would likely have the benefits of a very differentiated or heterogeneous gene code. The more varied your code, the more likely you are to survive a wide range of challenges or "attacks" from the environment. The more differentiated your gene code, the more likely you are to be an attractive individual. Attractiveness is just the outside manifestation or phenotype that signals to others that this person is healthy, well, and a possessor of good genes.

Is Beauty an Ideal Manufactured by Western Media?

Naomi Wolf, a controversial but well-respected feminist, author, speaker, and thinker argues in her book *The Beauty Myth* that ideals of beauty are created by advertising executives and other men in suits. She believes that women are enslaved to these contrived, often unattainable standards and feel bad about themselves because they can't measure up. She argues that:

> Women are mere 'beauties' in men's culture so that culture can be kept male. When women in culture show character, they are not desirable. A beautiful heroine is a contradiction in terms, since heroism is about individuality, interesting and ever changing, while 'beauty' is generic, boring, and inert. A cultural fixation on female thinness is not an obsession about female beauty but an obsession about female obedience. (Wolf, 2002)

This argument seems to be debunked, however, by studies that babies as young as two months can identify beauty (Langlois & Roggman, 1990; Langlois et al., 1987; Langlois, Roggman & Rieser-Danner, 1990). Furthermore, in an often-cited study, remote Indian tribes of Venezuela and Paraguay, who have never been exposed to Western media, were asked to evaluate and rate the beauty of Western women (Jones & Hill, 1993). The local Indians found the same characteristics beautiful as individuals questioned from Brazil, Russia and the U.S.

He's Gotta Have It: A major international study found that women everywhere desired and placed significant importance on "good financial prospects."

Each of these cultures associated female beauty with symmetry, small chins and large eyes—all character traits of youth and fertility. While the advertising tycoons of Madison Avenue are good, they aren't *that* good!

Male beauty has also been studied across cultures. In a comprehensive study of over 10,000 people from 37 cultures, women desired and placed significant importance on "good financial prospects." They valued qualities linked to resource acquisition such as ambition, industriousness, social status and older age (Buss, 1989). These consistencies were also seen in a study of Chinese, Indian and English women judging Greek men (Thakerar & Iwawaki, 1979). Across the world, it is obvious that these traits are consistently important for male attractiveness.

When an ethnically diverse group of college students were asked to judge the attractiveness of women from Asia, Europe, America, the Caribbean, and Latin America in photographs, they had strikingly similar findings (Cunningham, Roberts, Barbee, Druen & Wu, 1995). Despite the fact that these raters were racially and culturally diverse, they consistently identified the same facial traits as attractive, as well as the overall attractiveness ratings of the women. The raters preferred smaller noses, larger eyes that were further apart, petite chins, larger cheekbones, larger lower lips, expressive higher brows, dilated pupils, large smiles, and full hair.

The authors also wanted to evaluate the similarities or differences between black and white American men in regard to facial appearance and body preference in women. They asked black and white male college students to judge the appearance of photos of black college-age women. In addition, the volunteers were asked to indicate the ideal height and weight of a female and their favorite part of the female body. The black and white men's responses were exactly the same when it came to what they found attractive in women's facial features. However, they did differ in body preferences. The black men preferred a heavier female with larger buttocks.

Why do African and African-American Men Prefer Women with Big Butts?

What you goin' do with all that junk?
All that junk inside your trunk?
I'maget, get, get, get you drunk,
Get you love drunk off my hump.
—Black Eyed Peas, "My Humps"

Regardless of the culture, all males tend to prefer a curvy female. In Western society, men's magazines like *Playboy* and *Maxim* always feature curvaceous cover models with large breasts and hips. Not surprisingly, the desire for a well-proportioned, curvy female is common to other cultures and has been for centuries. However, in countries that are resource poor such as parts of Africa and Central America, a heavier female is considered more attractive than a thin one (Anderson, Crawford, Nadeau & Lindberg, 1992; Furnham & Baguma, 1994).

This contrasts with Westernized, resource-ample, or wealthier societies in which thinner females are found to be more desirable. The key factor in all cultures, regardless of the preferred weight, is the ideal waist-to-hip ratio of 0.7, or a waist that is thirty percent

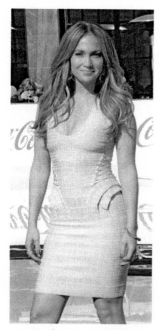

Jennifer Lopez is known for not only her singing and acting talent but also for her sexy figure.

smaller than the hips. In cultures that are poorer, a female with more fat subconsciously signals to a male that she can provide food for a baby and is genetically fit to be a good mate. A primary site where females store and show their fat is the buttocks, and this is one of the reasons why a larger behind has evolved to be recognized as very attractive in certain cultures.

Plumpness, or roundness, as well as a jutting backside are pervasive images in the traditional Nigerian African construct of female beauty. An ancient Yoruba proverb from Nigeria says, "Ours is ours, even if our child does not possess rounded buttocks, we would not therefore wear beads on the buttocks of someone else's daughter." This strongly suggests that a lot of cultural value is placed on a female's protruding backside (Oloruntoba-Oju, 2007). What you may find surprising is that this desire for females with larger buttocks is then ingrained into the culture for generations, regardless of moving to a more amply endowed society (Cunningham, et al., 1995).

The attraction to a full-figured, rounded backside is also found in many Latin American countries. I recently spoke about my beauty philosophies to a room of 350 plastic surgeons in Florianopolis, Brazil. While there, I had a wonderful opportunity to learn more about the cultural attitude toward cosmetic medicine and female body image. I was surprised by the greater emphasis the Latin American physicians placed on developing and offering enhancements of the hips, thighs, buttocks and waist area. They basically paid a lot more attention to the lower half of the body than we do in the U.S., as this is what they believe meets with their patients' desires. And each afternoon following the end of discussions, I would go for a run as I always do on my fact-finding exploration of a new country. I didn't have to go far to witness the cultural beauty differences between Brazil and the United States—all it took was a jog along the beach. You can't help but recognize the stark contrast in the style of Brazilian bikinis to those north of the equator. In Brazil, the prevailing style of bikini bottoms allows a majority of the junk in the trunk to be exposed, whereas the tops unceremoniously draw little or no attention. This is strikingly

> The Male Eye for Curves: The key factor in all cultures, regardless of the preferred weight, is the ideal waist-to-hip ratio of 0.7, or a waist that is thirty percent smaller than the hips.

different from the U.S., where bikini tops are Band-Aid size and the bottoms leave more room for the imagination.

My observations confirmed what the Brazilian doctors mentioned. And it's not surprising that the breast implant business in Brazil, although large, is significantly smaller both in the number of procedures performed and the average size of implants used as compared to the U.S. The trunk may be full in Latin America, but the cupboard is barely filled.

Therefore, it appears that there are a few basic physical characteristics that all populations find to be associated with attractiveness, regardless of race or culture. However, the manner in which each of these cultures emphasize and highlight the critical physical traits of beauty is different, which explains the world's variety of cultural difference in adornments, styles and expressions. Just as all cultures have slight differences in the foods they enjoy, they also share some basic similarities; nobody likes spoiled food regardless of their background.

Body Art: Piercing, Deformation, and Tattooing

Abraham's servant gave a golden earring of half a shekel weight and ten bracelets to Rebekah (Genesis 24:22).

From ancient times to the present, body piercing and tattooing have been practiced all over the world. The Old Testament refers to earrings and our earliest records of tattooing begin with the oldest mummified body discovered near the Italian Alps, Ötzi the Iceman, dated to 3300 BCE, who had a pierced ear and tattoos on his lower back.

Today, piercings are very popular in Western culture, as well as in Asia and Africa. Developing to become a symbol of adornment within each culture—modifying the ancient tradition and morphing it to fit within their own style—piercing likely began as a way for humans to highlight health and vitality. Men used piercings to signify to females and others that they were strong, resilient, and had the necessary resources to tolerate injury, much like how a man with battle scars is considered tested, tougher and sexier.

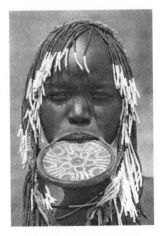

Piercings can also be used to highlight physical traits that exemplify femininity. Ethiopian women of the Mursi tribe place a large clay disc within the lip (lip plating), which is found to be attractive. While in America we don't see this as remotely attractive, it is just as unlikely that the Congo and East Africans find the collagen-filled female lips of Western women attractive. Both cultures,

Lip plating accentuates the sexuality of the lips.

> "I don't know who invented high heel shoes, but all women owe him a lot."
> —Marilyn Monroe

however, are trying to emphasize the same trait, a fuller lip, and are therefore highlighting a basic and universal female symbolism of fertility and youthfulness.

In ancient China, women bound their feet to the point of deformation. These women could barely walk on their mangled, miniaturized feet, but this was considered highly erotic to men. Why was such a seemingly tortuous act and unusual-appearing foot found attractive? By making a woman more helpless, this physical feature indicated youthfulness. For a female, the more directionally youthful a physical feature, the greater its beautifying value. In the paternalistic ancient Chinese culture, a childlike woman was considered attractive. But is Western culture so different? The five-inch heels considered erotic to many males in Western cultures are probably viewed by East Asian cultures as equally bizarre. The pumps and stilettos have the benefit of raising the buttocks in the air, theoretically presenting itself for a man. However,

similarly to Chinese foot binding, it also impairs a woman's ability to walk, making her appear a little more helpless. Like a foot-bound woman in ancient China, a modern American woman in five-inch heels could benefit from a strong man's assistance when crossing the room or the street, and men in all cultures like to feel needed by their mates.

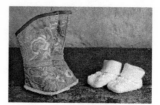

Why do people go through the pain of burning a permanent mark on their skin? Traditionally, to tolerate a tattoo you had to be pretty tough. It's a painful act and you better be healthy because someone who is weak or sick could be at risk for infection or worse. Soldiers returning from battle in a faraway land may come back with a tattoo to commemorate their experience and symbolize heroism as well. In some sub-Saharan African cultures it is still popular to this day to scar faces, backs and arms by branding the skin with hot pokers, sticks and hooks. The marks create fabulous designs that have enormous religious or cultural significance or are chosen simply for aesthetic purposes.

Tattooing, similarly to piercing, still symbolizes strength, maturity, and the ability to tolerate injury, and it's considered attractive in many African societies. While for a long time tattooing or scarification was once frowned upon or deemed sacrilegious in the West,

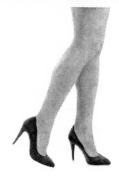

Like the Chinese tradition of foot binding, which continued even after it was banned in 1912, modern-day spike heels render women somewhat helpless, signaling that they could use a strong man's assistance.

tattooing is now found in 36% of Americans ages 18–29, 24% of those 30-40 and 15% of those 41-51 (Laumann & Derick, 2006). Artistic, proud, and loud ink designs are etched into the skin, and like traditional African tattoos, the ink may symbolize something in the culture or be chosen to beautify one's appearance. Our modern day actions link us to African and historical counterparts a world away.

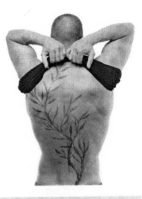

Who's So Vain?

While today it is very commonplace for Americans to dye their hair, it was once considered vain and shrouded in secrecy. In the early twentieth century, Americans attached a stigma to hair coloring, and it was not until a Clairol advertising campaign in the 1950s that asked, "Did she or didn't she?" that the stigma began to dissolve. But even then, only about seven percent of Americans colored their hair (Sherrow, 2006). Eventually, due in part to the erosion of the stigma and marketing efforts that urged people to cover gray or "have more fun" as a blonde, the number of Americans who dye their hair steadily rose from forty percent in the 1970s to over seventy-five percent today.

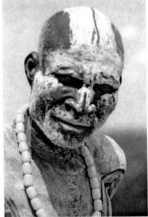

Tattooing, like scarification and piercing, enhances attractiveness because it symbolizes strength, maturity, and the ability to tolerate injury.

Does that make us vainer than our parents or grandparents? Vanity is a relative term that's only definable within the context of the society in which it's discussed. What one culture may find vain, another considers mainstream. When I first started giving Botox treatments in the late 1990s, they were a secret that many were hesitant to reveal to their friends. The shame didn't last long and by early 2000, Botox parties were commonplace. Groups of women and men got together to enjoy fun, food and friends while their accommodating neighborhood cosmetic doctor/ nurse treated them with Botox. (Today this practice is discouraged and regarded as ethically questionable by most academic medical societies in the U.S.) In puritanical cultures, altering the face with surgery may seem to violate religion, an attitude based on scriptures such as, "The Lord does not look at the things man looks at. Man looks at the outward appearance, but the Lord looks at the heart" (Samuel 16:7). But in parts of South America, plastic surgery is so widespread and commonplace that people wear bandages like a badge of honor.

The human urge to beautify ourselves is not restricted by age, time or space. Across all millennia, cultures and religions, people have found socially acceptable ways to beautify themselves. From simple acts of brushing hair to complex surgical breast implants, the desire to highlight female sexually traits and appear attractive is a natural human urge that is consistent throughout nature. It only varies in how each society chooses to manifest it.

In Iran, where it's common to wear a burqa that covers most of a woman's face except for her nose and eyes, rhinoplasty (nose reshaping) is the number-one cosmetic surgical procedure. And in a socially liberal society like the U.S., where body-revealing styles including thong bathing suits, miniskirts and silk dresses are common, liposuction is the most popular plastic surgical procedure. The measures we go through to appear attractive may be different as seen in the adornments, facial or body features each culture chooses to emphasize, but we are all connected by the raw sense of what we define as physically beautiful. Across all cultures, men universally want mates younger than themselves (Buss, 1989). However, the status of the female's virginity varies by culture. Men from China, India and Iran place tremendous value on virginity, but those from Scandinavian countries and the Netherlands put little importance on chastity.

Where We're Headed

In which part of the world do you think beauty is the most important factor in choosing a mate: Nigeria, Europe, Zambia, the U.S. or India? As obsessed as American culture seems to be with youth and beauty, Nigeria, Zambia and India place more emphasis on physical attraction in selecting a partner than Europe or North America. As surprising as it may sound, cultures with the highest levels of disease rate attractiveness as more important; in the less developed nations, where resources are in short supply, both sexes tend to place more emphasis on appearance (Gangestad & Buss, 1993). From an evolutionary perspective, this makes sense. In resource-depleted countries, one's physical exterior may be the best way to identify health and genetic fitness. In a wealthy country with a greater chance of more people reaching their genetic potential, appearance is not as valuable and other criteria of attractiveness gain increasing importance. This is an indication of the evolutionary direction our species is taking. As society modernizes, being artistic, musical, humorous and having other talents that indicate intelligence will become more important criteria in choosing a mate (Miller, 2008).

CHAPTER 8

IS HE OR ISN'T SHE?

"Male gorillas court and couple with each other, grizzly bear families have two mothers; male swans form pair-bonds with one another. . . . The world is, indeed, teeming with homosexual, bisexual and transgendered creatures of every stripe and feather."

—from *Biological Exuberance: Animal Homosexuality and Natural Diversity* by Bruce Bagemihl

A couple I was very friendly with for many years got divorced not long ago, which amazed me because their marriage seemed to be pretty solid. Although they were never affectionate to each other, the two of them got along very well and seemed the best of friends, which is probably where the problem lay. The husband had recently come out and admitted that he was gay and was moving to Europe to be with another man. When I last talked to him, he told me that he always knew he was gay, but fought it for many years because he was afraid to succumb to it. After decades of living a lie, he now feels free and is much happier because he is being true to himself.

After hearing his story, I came to learn that this situation isn't that uncommon. It's estimated that somewhere between 1.7 to 3.4 million American women are married to men who have sex with other men (Laumann, 1990). I know several other couples that have split, sometimes after more than twenty years of marriage, because either the husband or wife conceded to his or her attraction to the same sex. In each case, they said they had

119

always known about their sexual preference but didn't want to face it and/or suppressed it to avoid hurting their children or other members of their family. The question begs to be answered were they born gay or did something cause them to develop attraction to the same sex.

> Thanks to less dogmatism, our scientific understanding of homosexuality's origins and impact is gaining strength.

From ancient Greek and Roman societies to modern-day American, European, and African cultures, homosexuality has been prevalent throughout recorded history. What was once listed as a psychopathology in the American Psychiatry Association Diagnostic and Statistical Manual of Mental Disorder (DSM–I) is now considered by many as a genetic destiny. In the footsteps of the Kinsey Report, a robust gay rights movement, and changing societal attitudes, homosexuality's pathological label was revoked in 1973 when it was removed from the DSM. But regardless of its label, there is no denying that homosexuality is a socially and politically laden issue. Even the scientists who try to study it objectively must be sensitive to their own biases when evaluating its origins, boundaries, and impact on society.

For many years, it was rather easy to put human sexuality into a neatly defined box of either gay or straight. However, issues such as HIV, which are more prevalent within the male community practicing homosexual behaviors (both gay and straight), have forced science to take a bolder and more honest look at the sizable portion of the population that has feelings, sexual relations, and pairs with the same gender. Thanks to open-ended surveys and less dogmatism, the edges of what is and isn't homosexual have become blurred, and our understanding of its origins and impact are gaining strength.

How Common Is Being Gay?

(Reuters: October 10, 2007) - Addressing New York's Columbia University last month, President Mahmoud Ahmadinejad replied to a question about gays in the Islamic Republic saying: "In Iran we don't have homosexuals like in your country."

Speaking through a translator, he also said: "In Iran we don't have this phenomenon."

Homosexuality is punishable by death in the Islamic Republic.

"What Ahmadinejad said was not a political answer. He said that, compared to American society, we don't have many homosexuals," presidential media adviser Mohammad Kalhor said.

Kalhor told Reuters that because of historical, religious and cultural differences homosexuality was less common in Iran and the Islamic world than in the West.

Despite the Iranian President's comments, the general consensus is that about ten percent of the human population is homosexual, but different definitions of homosexuality may alter this number. Alfred Kinsey, one of the first to take on the challenge of defining sexuality, believed we're all on a spectrum of zero to six, with six being exclusively homosexual and zero being exclusively heterosexual. However, he believed most people fall somewhere in between these extremes with occasional homosexual tendencies, fantasies, and perhaps occasional sexual acts in the presence of others of the same sex, but realizing that only a small proportion of those who experience homosexual acts actually adopt gay or lesbian identities. So, while studies quote homosexual acts as high as twenty-six percent in the populations (Kinsey, Pomeroy & Martin, 2010), the actual incidence of those who define themselves as homosexual in Western culture likely ranges from five to twelve percent (Sell, Wells & Wypij, 1995). In another survey of contemporary American women, up to seventeen percent have had homosexual sex, but only five percent considered themselves gay or bisexual (Janus & Janus, 1993).

When this much of the population is experiencing same gender sexual relations and it doesn't result in procreation, the Darwinian evolutionist in us looks for the reason why such a behavior exists at all.

Evolution doesn't make mistakes.

If homosexuality had a negative effect on our species' adaptation, we would expect it to be "stomped out." However, homosexuality is prevalent with humans, and moreover, we see homosexual behavior and pairing in other primates such as pygmy chimpanzees and gorillas (Parish, 1994; White, 1989). Therefore, homosexual behavior must have a beneficial effect on our species and society.

> Because of its prevalence, homosexual behavior must have a beneficial effect on our species and society— one theory suggests that a gay family member conserves family resources by helping care for nieces and nephews and not depleting resources with his/her own family.

Anthropologists are still debating what that beneficial effect might be, and how it all began. One prevailing theory says that homosexuality aids in kinship—in a family with multiple siblings, it would be best if one of the extra males or females was homosexual so he or she could help raise his/her nieces and nephews and not further deplete resources with his/her own additional family. This argument is supported by the fact that homosexuality is more common as we go lower in the birth order. In other words, the later a son is born in a family, the more likely he is to be gay. Self-identified male homosexuals in the U.S. and Canada tend to have more older brothers than do self-identified heterosexuals (Blanchard & Bogaert, 1996). And historically, the Lache of Colombia and in societies of the West Indies, sons of low birth orders were at times raised as daughters (Greenberg, 1988; Metraux & Kirchoff, 1948).

The general consensus is that about ten percent of the population is gay.

Another explanation, the parental manipulation theory, says that it would be beneficial to parents with multiple children to have one child who is homosexual so that the gay child can help in raising siblings or the offspring of siblings instead of devoting their energy and resources to starting their own family. Parental manipulation of a child to be homosexual may also aid the family's social, political, or religious status. From politically motivated families in fifteenth-century Florence to the castrated Eunuchs of the Byzantine courts and transgender shamans of South America, parents have encouraged their children into homosexual behavior throughout history. But for these theories to be supported there should ultimately be evidence of better survival and greater reproductive success in families with homosexuals. However, this data is weak or unfounded at this time.

Don't Ask, Don't Tell

In 1993, President Bill Clinton, a pragmatist in many ways, had to search for a diplomatic solution to whether or not gays should or could be admitted into the military. There has always been an undercurrent of discrimination against openly gay men and women in the military—mostly for homophobic reasons, perhaps. But many cultural and military leaders felt that openly gay soldiers "would create an unacceptable risk to the high standards of morale, good order and discipline, and unit cohesion that are the essence of military capability."

Gays are represented in higher numbers in the military than in the general population.

However, all the military brass would have to do is review the history of militaries world over to realize that gays have often been part of the military and in fact are represented in higher numbers in these forces than in the general population. And there is some reason to believe that they are better equipped and positioned to be soldiers as well. Faced with a split legislature, President Clinton came up with his famously ambiguous "Don't Ask, Don't Tell" policy.

Under this system, the military will not ask you to reveal if you're gay, and in return you are not obligated to tell the military if you are, and then everything is OK. If you however, openly act out or admit you are gay then you can be barred from service. Hmm . . . I wonder how people the world over would like it if governments made compromises like "Don't Ask, Don't Tell" for something like, say, paying taxes. I know my kids would love such a policy when it comes to cleaning their rooms or answering for who ate the last cookie from the cookie jar. In 2011, "Don't Ask, Don't Tell" was repealed, and openly gay men and women are now allowed into the military.

The military issues involving homosexuality may become even less controversial if one increasingly popular theory takes hold. The theory about homosexuality that seems to be gaining the most support with academics is called reciprocal altruism, or alliance formation. This implies that homosexuality results in forging strong alliances between individuals of the same gender, which in turn can help secure resources. When a society gets to the point that investing in the already born rather than creating more offspring provides greater benefit to the population, same-sex alliances would be selectively adaptive and beneficial to the society. Too many offspring may drain resources, whereas homosexual alliances can be helpful to gather and defend resources. Therefore, homosexuality is not a reproductive strategy, but rather a survival strategy. Men that form close bonds are better equipped to defend, as evidenced by the fifty-percent greater likelihood of homosexual behavior in the military than in a random civilian population (Fay, Turner, Klassen & Gagnon, 1989). In addition, benefits of lesbian relationships in helping negotiate alliances, extend trade networks and build economic security can be seen in some native African societies (Blackwood, 1986).

> Another prominent theory states that homosexuality allows the forging of strong alliances that help the community gather and defend resources.

This theory doesn't take into account sexual acts of pleasure, and certainly many men and women can forge strong alliances without having sexual relations. But regardless of orientation, sex is used to solidify bonds and keep people close. Sex, therefore, adds more to a relationship than just procreation. In fact, in humans and in some other primates such as the pygmy chimpanzees, sexual acts are rarely conceptive. And because sexual relations are pleasurable, when two people want to strengthen and maintain a relationship, it's intuitive that sexual acts would become a part of the relationship bond. The reciprocal altruism theory would then explain close friends of the same gender who occasionally engage in sexual acts at convenient time periods or for political and/or social gain.

> Regardless of orientation, sex is used to solidify bonds and keep people close.

Such behavior is rather common in other primates and can be observed in humans as well. In fact, the data proves that most people who report engaging in a homosexual act are not self-identified as gay. Some academics believe reciprocal altruism explains homosexual behavior as a form of friendship or socialization and not at all on the same spectrum of conceptive heterosexuality. This explains how a person can engage in homosexual acts with a close friend, as all friendships have close bonds and occasionally may be acted on but still be a heterosexual (De Block & Adriaens, 2004). While such theories can neatly explain bisexuality, it doesn't account for exclusive homosexuality.

Still Asking: Nature or Nurture?

Are people who are exclusively homosexual and self-identified gay born that way, or do they choose to be gay?

This is a very hotly debated issue with political ramifications. Certainly, if people can choose to be gay, they can choose not to be.

For many years, being gay was thought to be a lifestyle choice and one that could be reversed by psychotherapy or exorcism. Freud, who was quite controversial in his discussions on homosexuality, suggested there was a psychological component stemming from early in life. He believed that arrests in sexual development might lead to angst and repressions that become manifested later in life in sexual dysfunction or unusual behaviors (Dean & Lane, 2001). While Freud believed homosexuality to be a perversion, he didn't think it was necessarily a sickness. In fact, he felt homosexuality was only a pathological problem when it was repressed, in which case it could lead to neuroses. However, in his well-documented 1935 letter written to a mother concerned about her son's homosexuality, Freud's reassurance that homosexuality was nothing to be ashamed of and that many of history's greatest leaders were gay—from Plato to Michelangelo to DaVinci—supports his view that homosexuality was not a disease to cure, but a variant of the normal that doesn't need addressing unless causing psychological disturbances (Abelove, 2005). And although he had multiple theories on the specific childhood experiences that lead to homosexual behaviors, Freud was open to the possibility that homosexuality is organically pre-determined (De Block & Adriaens, 2004).

> Freud thought homosexuality was not a disease to be cured but a variant of the normal—unless it was repressed and led to neurotic behavior such as being overly tense or anxious.

In today's terms, this would be called being genetically predisposed to homosexuality. The genetic disposition explanation is fueling the prevailing winds of conventional wisdom, and fortunately leading to a greater acceptance of gay people by the majority. And it is a politically favorable view, because it recuses blame and has the potential to lead to less discrimination.

In contrast, believing that homosexuality is a result of a "gay gene" also creates an opening for a eugenic route to discrimination. The Nazis' delusions of grandeur about a master race launched a mission to stamp out undesirable genes, and in their deranged philosophy, homosexual behavior was to be expunged from the population.

> Genetics has some impact on being gay, but it's not the whole story.

Half a century later, we still debate the nature versus nurture origin of homosexuality. In a Gallup Poll, the amount of people in the U.S. that believed homosexuality was inborn tripled from 1977 to 2001, from thirteen to forty percent (Sheldon, Pfeffer, Jayaratne, Feldbaum, & Petty, 2007).

However, if homosexuality were all due to genetics, you would have to assume that two people who share the exact same genes would likely have the same sexual orientation.

Scientists test such ideas in twin studies. Monozygotic, or identical twins, share the same exact genetic information. Identical twin studies reveal that when one twin is a non-heterosexual, fifty-two percent of the time the other one is also non-heterosexual, for fraternal or non-identical twins who do share the exact same genetic information, the chance of the second one also being non-heterosexual is twenty-two percent. For brothers where one is gay, the likelihood of a non-twin related brother also being non-heterosexual is nine percent (J. M. Bailey & Pillard, 1991). This data shows that genetics has some impact on being non-heterosexual, but it cannot be the whole story because two people with the same exact genetic material are not always both gay. Therefore, environment has to have some impact on whether or not it is expressed or acted upon.

How's Your Gaydar?

Did you know about Ricky Martin all along?

In 2010, the singer publicly acknowledged for the first time that he is gay. "I am proud to say that I am a fortunate homosexual man. I am very blessed to be who I am," he said in a statement, finally revealing one of the worst kept secrets in music.

He had assiduously hid his sexuality early in his career, when he was a member of the Latin boy band Menudo. But once he went solo 1991 and broke through with his first album in English, which contained the hit "Livin' la Vida Loca," his sexuality became increasingly evident. He seemed to be much more open in his mannerisms and choice of partners as his career blossomed, but he never explicitly acknowledged being gay. In 2008, Martin had twin sons, Valentino and Mateo, via a surrogate, and he dropped out of the limelight to be a dad.

Martin grew up in a Catholic home in Puerto Rico and was an altar boy until he joined Menudo. The Catholic Church condemns homosexuality, which may explain partly why he professed his love for Mexican TV hostess Rebecca de Alba, and the two shared an off-and-on-again relationship for more than fourteen years. In 2000 he was asked point-blank during an interview with the UK newspaper *The Mirror* to address rumors about his sexuality, and he firmly denied being gay. "I guess these rumors were started by people who don't have a life, or perhaps it's because they want me to be like them and I'm not," he said. It would take another decade for him to reveal his true self (*The Improper*, 2010).

Can you tell if someone is gay by the way they look? In order to answer that question, there has to be a stereotype of what a gay person looks like. For gay males, that stereotype would be a more feminine appearance, and for lesbians, a more masculine appearance. Scientists recognize this phenomenon as gender inversion, and prior to the twentieth century, before the word "homosexuality" was coined or "gay" or "lesbian" were the

Before the words "homosexual," "gay" or "lesbian" were the common vernacular, gays were known as "gender inverts."

common vernacular, those who we would think of today of as gay were known as "gender inverts." In other words, homosexual men were considered psychologically women and homosexual women psychologically men, and therefore were thought to act and have the same preferences of their adopted gender. Extending this reasoning and labeling these individuals as gender inverts would make them appear more like the opposite sex. The question becomes, is there any truth to gender inversion appearance? Do gay men look feminine and gay women look masculine, and can we detect this from video or photographic evaluation only?

This has been studied, and judgments by unknowing observers reviewing ten-second videos of both gay and straight individuals relied more heavily on body motion than body appearance when judging sexual orientation. Moreover, their judgments were accurate above chance (Rieger, Linsenmeier, Gygax, Garcia & Bailey, 2010; Rieger, Linsenmeier, Gygax & Bailey, 2008).

Homosexual behaviors and motions could certainly be learned and adopted, but how about simple appearance? Could you tell if people are gay by just looking at a photo of their face?

In a 2010 study, male faces that were morphed to appear more feminine and female faces that were morphed to appear more masculine were likely to be judged as gay (Freeman, Johnson, Ambady & Rule, 2010). When researchers followed this up with real photos of gay and straight men and women and asked participants to judge the faces for their level of masculinity, femininity, and sexual orientation, the judges were more likely than chance to accurately identify the people in the photos as gay or straight. However, the judges were also wrong forty-two percent of the time by incorrectly judging a gay person straight, and twenty-two percent of the time by judging a straight person gay. What was interesting is that gender inversion cues influence perceptions of sexual orientation. The more feminine a man or more masculine a woman appears, the more likely an unknowing observer would correctly identify him or her as gay. The accuracy certainly increases when you add gait, motion, and speech, all which provide clues of sexual orientation and strong evidence that there really is such a thing as "Gaydar."

> The more feminine a man or more masculine a woman appears, the more likely an unknowing observer would correctly identify him or her as gay.

Appearance — Do Gays Really Care More?

This question has been posed by many. Gay men are often referred to as "neat" or "particular" and lesbians are thought to be less concerned and willing to accept all body types. The science shows that yes, gay men do seem to be somewhat more concerned about their appearance than heterosexuals and more likely to be affected by body image disorders. While lesbianism seems to buffer against body image distortion to some extent, the jury is still out, as some studies have also suggested that lesbians are likely subjected to and fall suspect to the same image pressures as their heterosexual contemporaries (Peplau et al., 2009).

In the U.S., eight percent of those who get cosmetic procedures are men (American Society of Aesthetic Plastic Surgery, 2011). While this organization doesn't determine if they are gay or not, the percentage closely mirrors the gay population proportion in the U.S. Although we often hear from media outlets about the rise in men getting plastic surgery, it has been my experience that the number of men getting plastic surgery remains pretty much flat and seems to be similar to the consistency in homosexuality rates. Over the eleven years I've been in practice, the proportion of men seeking my services for cosmetic procedures has not gone up significantly.

However, one area in which being gay has had an intimate association with plastic surgery over the last decade is the HIV patient who suffers from facial fat atrophy, or "facial wasting." The protease inhibitor medications that are helpful to keeping the HIV virus at bay also may result in a loss of fat in the face. The face of these individuals greatly thins and the skeletal structures become accentuated. This facial wasting appearance is highly correlated with HIV status, and for men it can be a tell-tale sign that they harbor the HIV virus. Many gay men (and even some who are not gay, but are cognizant of this condition) are highly sensitive and self-conscious of this appearance because they believe it leads to discrimination. In plastic surgery, the last decade has seen great advancements in developing solutions to improving their appearance. We can use office-based filler treatments to volumize their faces to replace lost fullness in areas that have been depleted from fat loss. One of these filler products, Sculptra™, uses micronized particles to stimulate collagen formation in the skin and tissues below. In an office-based procedure that takes only minutes, the product is injected into the skin approximately three times over a six week period, and the face starts to gradually fill in. The correction can be expected to last for eighteen months. The face gains a healthier appearance and of course, the patients' disposition changes soon after. The FDA recognizing the safety, efficacy, and benefits of this product for HIV patients, and gave its approval in 2004. The manufacturer enacted a special cost-saving program that allows HIV patients reduced pricing, making it more widely available for a larger part of the gay population.

> The safety, efficacy, and benefits of a product that corrects the gaunt features that accompany some HIV medications led to the product's FDA approval a few years ago.

Soon after Sculptra's approval, Radiesse, another filler product, received FDA approval for treating HIV patients. However, Radiesse offered immediate same-day correction. For the HIV patient, this was a great success, but there is a subset of my non-HIV patients who also suffer from facial wasting. Many marathon runners and those who exercise heavily may experience loss of fat from their faces. They too want to be treated. Additionally, during the normal aging processes, many people experience natural atrophy and want a filling of their faces. Soon, these filler products were being used off label to treat many people, both HIV and non-HIV, for cosmetic use. Today, Scultptra and Radiesse are popular products for rejuvenating the aging face. However, although rare, there are some risks that should be recognized and it is important to see an experienced practitioner. If not injected appropriately, the treatment could have disfiguring results.

My practice also treats many gay men who are interested in feminizing their features. Hair is a sexually dimorphic trait and to remove all of one's hair is generally a feminizing act. Today, bare torsos are fashionable, and we're seeing an increasing amount of non-gay men asking to have their chest, back, and pubic hair removed. Additional feminizing procedures commonly requested by our gay male patients include enlarging lips with fillers. Moreover, while Botox is popular in both our gay and straight male population, more than ten percent of the men we treat in my practice are gay. The lesbian women we treat don't ask for masculinizing procedures, but rather are interested in the same feminizing procedures as straight women.

Born In the Wrong Body

I recently saw a woman in consultation who wanted a nasal reshaping procedure. A tall lady at about six-foot two, with long hair, painted nails and large breasts, she also had some masculine-looking facial and hand features. Her nose was large, twisted, out of proportion to the rest of her face, and not at all feminine. She asked to have it made more aesthetically pleasing, but not too much of a change, and most importantly she wanted to be able to breathe through it well. I reviewed her medical history as did my physician assistant. When asked about any previous surgeries, she didn't say anything about having undergone sexual reassignment surgery. At the time of her nasal surgery it was confirmed she had undergone surgical treatments to alter her natural genital anatomy. This is not the first time a transgender person has refrained from mentioning or hiding his or her previous procedures. Although it's uncommon for us to not find out until the time of surgery—usually we come to a mutual understanding prior to the procedure—it seems to me that some transsexual people are so convinced in their psyche that they are the opposite gender that they naturally repress admitting they've had reassignment surgery.

> Transsexuals are so convinced in their psyche that they are the opposite gender that they naturally repress admitting they've had reassignment surgery.

Gender reassignment surgery, in which females are surgically altered to represent males or males to be female, is beyond the scope of this book, but it is worth a mention because plastic surgery is so intimately necessary to the process. Reassignment surgery can include, but is not limited to, facial plastic surgery, vocal cord surgery, and genital reassignment surgery. Those who undergo the surgery are generally known as transsexual, or the more recent term, possessing a gender identity disorder. They do not believe they are gay, but rather that they were born trapped in the wrong body type. In fact, studies have shown that they may have brain morphology or brain structures similar to the opposite sex (Kruijver et al., 2000; Zhou, Hofman, Gooren & Swaab, 1995). Gender dysphoria, or distress resulting from conflicting gender identity, and sex assignment are rarities, approximately one out of every 30,000 men and one out of every 100,000 women will seek gender reassignment surgery (Landén, Wålinder & Lundström, 1996).

I see transgender male to female patients in my practice who are mostly interested in maintaining their feminizing attributes with products such as wrinkle reducers, fillers, and lasers. Many times, the combination of hormone therapy and plastic surgery are done so effectively that it becomes difficult on first glance to determine physically their natal sex or to what gender they were born. Many of the transgender patients who openly express, or "come out" and live as they wish, find that they lead a much more authentic life, gain self-confidence, and experience less depression and improved communication (Alegria & University of Nevada, 2008).

Unfortunately, HIV is more commonly found in the transgender population, and these people also experience greater rates of unemployment, discrimination, ridicule and suicide (Clements-Nolle, Marx, Guzman & Katz, 2001; Clements-Nolle, Marx & Katz, 2006; Fitzpatrick, Euton, Jones & Schmidt, 2005; Kenagy, 2005). In order to emotionally prepare gender identity patients prior to undergoing gender reassignment surgery, most clinics require at least one to two years of psychotherapy and one year of living as the opposite gender.

The more we learn, the more we can move forward with ourselves and each other.

Homosexuality appears in a large part of all populations and is natural to all societies. Regardless of its origin or meaning, same sex pairing will always be part of our world. Its only significance to plastic surgery is that there really is no significance—people gain improved self-esteem through positive changes in their appearance regardless of their gender preference.

Nature thrives on diversity. And people of all persuasions achieve their highest potential when they're honest with themselves and others.

CHAPTER 9

DO-IT-YOURSELF
ALLURE

"The best thing is to look natural, but it takes makeup to look natural."
—Calvin Klein

"I love the confidence that makeup gives me."
—Tyra Banks

Makeup has its origins as a camouflaging technique used by men during battle to frighten enemies or symbolize the status of chieftains. When it was adopted by women, it evolved into a tool for emphasizing feminine traits that cultures the world over consider beautiful. Makeup is ubiquitous in Western and many Eastern societies, making it big business. In the United States alone, the cosmetic and toiletries industry is worth about a $50 billion.

But exactly how does wearing makeup benefit women?

We decided to investigate the effects of cosmetics on women and society in order to better understand why women wear them. In a 2007 study evaluating the effects makeup had on the first impression one projects, we enrolled women to have makeup applied by a professional makeup artist. Standardized photos were taken before and after the application. Then both photos for each subject were divided into four books with each subject represented in each book only once. Unknowing volunteer raters were then asked to complete a survey of questions for two of the books. Raters were unaware that the women in the photos had anything done and never saw the same person's photos twice. They were asked to rate the photos in the categories of social skills, academic performance, dating success, occupational success, attractiveness, financial success, relationship success, and athletic success. After our statistician evaluated all the responses, we were eager to find out if the women wearing makeup projected a better first impression. We discovered that in the categories of social skills, academic performance, and financial success, our raters found the makeup-wearing women projected a better first impression. In the categories of academic performance, financial success, and relationship success, those who were wearing makeup also had higher mean scores, although not statistically significant.

This study supports the theory that facial cosmetics can positively improve the first impression and the judgment others make about a woman.

Other trials have reported similar findings, showing that women who wear makeup appear to enjoy more prestigious jobs, greater earning potential, greater health, and more self-confidence (Nash, Fieldman, Hussey, Lévêque & Pineau, 2006). But do you think the women really have more self-confidence, or do they just look like they do? According to many studies and anecdotal findings, women really do feel better about themselves after putting on makeup. Although most studies that find makeup benefits a woman's self-esteem are done on younger women, age doesn't seem to be a factor when it comes to makeup being important to feeling good about one's self. More mature, aged, and infirmed women who are in the hospital feel greater self-confidence and are more apt to participate in social activities if they put on makeup (Holme, Beattie & Fleming, 2002).

> Facial cosmetics can positively improve the first impression—many studies reveal that women really do feel better about themselves after putting on makeup.

Because of this, my team of estheticians (professionals who specialize in cosmetic skin care) frequently participate in programs in the hospital cancer ward or travel to assisted-living facilities to treat women to facial makeovers. It never ceases to amaze me how much happiness and joy the women who are very sick or hospitalized feel after having a makeover. It is only dwarfed by my amazement of those closed-minded individuals who feel that more mature or ill persons won't gain positive feelings from makeup and/or pampering. All one needs to do is spend one day with our aesthetic team in a nursing home to realize that applying makeup and being made to feel beautiful has an enormous impact on one's disposition. These women seem to brighten up, stand taller, and become more social. Makeup for women of all ages can result in elevated feelings of self-confidence and self-worth—two of humanity's most basic needs. We never stop wanting to looking better, and to deny this is to deny human nature.

The Real Ladies of Deerfield Place

My mom who could be the most selfless and generous person alive, is unfortunately afflicted with Multiple Sclerosis (MS), a chronic and progressively debilitating neurological condition. She lives in an assisted-living home with approximately 100 other individuals. She really enjoys the company of the other residents and often gets together with the other ladies for lunch and bridge. Entertainment is brought in once a week, but while always very appreciated, they don't always get the best acts. Occasionally, educational speakers or self-help professionals come in, which everyone also enjoys.

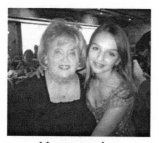

My mom and my oldest daughter, Ari.

Also once a week, many of the women who are more mobile get the opportunity to visit a nearby beauty shop to get their hair and nails done. It's obvious that many of the women look so very forward to this day, perhaps more so than any of the other activities. However, after talking to my mom, it became clear that many of the women who, like her, find it difficult to get out for the day of beautifying feel dispirited. These women, despite their infirmed condition and advanced age, still are very interested in looking their best. So my team of estheticians (skin care specialists) and I decided to bring beautifying treatments to them.

We arranged to have four of our estheticians travel north of the city to their complex and treat the ladies who desired a day of luxury. We set up the common room, where they normally play cards, into a mini day spa. Each lady was treated to a special facial, including a light peel, followed by a cosmetic makeover. Every forty-five minutes we would welcome in another lady. Following their treatment, you could not only see their excitement, pleasure, and gratitude, but feel it, too. It was a magical experience. At the end of the day I'm not sure who felt more special—the ladies we treated, or me and my staff.

The placement of makeup causes many women to enjoy an elevated self-esteem which translates into a physical manifestation that is favorably perceived by others and can significantly enhance a woman's image (Nash et al., 2006). Therefore, makeup is a powerful tool in a woman's arsenal for gaining advantage.

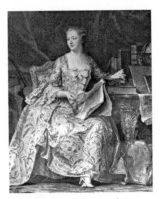

Madame Pompadour

At times, this advantage has been surrounded in controversy. What was once a well-accepted practice during the Egyptian dynasty became maligned in Medieval Europe. In the fourteenth through eighteenth centuries, rouge and dark red lipstick were considered the stuff of prostitutes. For the most part, makeup was vilified and considered not becoming of a lady and insulting to the Lord. Yet, this didn't stop women from using it. After receiving her last rites from her priest, Madame Pompadour put rouge on her face, and then died.

English Parliament, fearful that makeup was a powerful enough tool for women to deceive men, banned cosmetics in the late eighteenth century with a formal declaration:

> *All women, of whatever age, rank, profession, or degree, whether virgins, maids, or widows, that shall, from and after such Act, impose upon, seduce, or betray into matrimony, any of his Majesty's male subjects by the scents, paints, cosmetic washes, artificial teeth, false hair, Spanish wool, iron stays, hoops, high-heeled shoes, etc., shall incur the penalty of the law now enforced against witchcraft and like misdemeanors, and that the marriage upon conviction shall stand null and void.*
>
> *(Corson, 1972)*

As the nineteenth century came to an end, rouge was still considered the face paint of prostitutes and other seedy individuals. However, despite being socially gauche, women still wanted to "paint," and they recognized that when done subtly, it could highlight feminine character traits. It was hard to suppress this urge to enhance one's attractiveness.

> Makeup raises self-esteem and is a powerful tool in a woman's arsenal for gaining advantage.

The cosmetic industry exploded in twentieth century America and marked the first time since ancient Egypt that the unlimited use of cosmetics came to be universally accepted both socially and morally. The U.S. population increased by twenty percent between 1900 and 1910, but sales of cosmetics increased 100 percent. This explosion in both population and willingness to accept cosmetics paved the way for American entrepreneurs who took cosmetics to the next level, including Max Factor (Maximilian Faktorowicz, 1877-1938), Helena Rubinstein (Chaja Rubinstein, 1870 -1965) and Elizabeth Arden (Florence Graham 1878-1966).

Today, more money is spent on beauty products than education or social services. The U.S. spends two times as much on personal care products and services as on reading materials. Worldwide cosmetics and toiletries are a $134 billion dollar industry, with the U.S. representing about thirty percent of the market.

On my quest to understand beauty the world over in late 2011, I took a pilgrimage to the Neues Museum in the former East Berlin to see for myself an artwork said to represent the prettiest woman to ever grace the earth. This masterpiece, thought to have been completed in the thirteenth century B.C. by the Egyptian sculptor Thutmose, is a life-size bust of Nefertiti, the wife of the Egyptian Pharaoh Akhenaten. The bust, created in Nefertiti's lifetime, was discovered in Egypt by German excavators in 1912 and was first put on display to the public in 1924. A holy relic to plastic surgeons, it was officially adopted as the symbol for the American Society of Aesthetic Plastic Surgeons, and many plastic surgeons from the world over make their way to Berlin to view arguably the most perfect and famous Egyptian artifact ever discovered. With its overwhelming facial

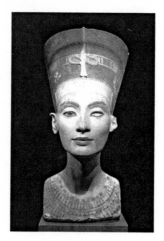

Nefertiti Bust

symmetry, idealized dimensions, and subtle but powerful femininity, the sculpture has become the iconic symbol of beauty the world over.

Words truly do not do it justice. The Nefertiti bust is one of the few pieces of art that I have found as good if not better than what I expected. As both an artist and plastic surgeon, I was captivated and enthralled by the aura of this famous face. The attention to detail and accuracy, from the tiniest folds of skin around the lips to the curved concavities around the eyes, indicates an artisan skilled in the science of beauty. From her makeup to her hinting smile, Nefertiti's image gives us a glimpse into a royal ancient Egyptian woman's psyche. It is almost as if Nefertiti is talking and her inner feelings are on display. The piece truly captures the essence of a woman and how the spirit can be projected in physical appearance. To this day, the image of Nefertiti and its impact on femininity is burned into my consciousness.

Makeup Strategies
Eyes

Nature's strategy for signaling feminine beauty starts with the eyes, where we communicate our interest and desires. For a woman, increasing the contrast between light-colored skin and darker eyes further reinforces her femininity.

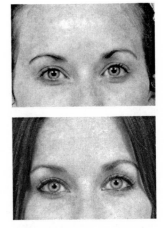

No one seems to exemplify beauty and this form of facial painting better than Nefertiti and Cleopatra, considered two of the most glamorous women to ever live and memorialized as the perfect beauties. They are portrayed in paintings and sculptures with deep, dark blue- and black-painted eye shadow and liner extending beyond the outside corners of the eyelids.

Increasing contrast between the eyes and surrounding skin further beautifies the eyes.

In addition to its use as a beautifier, makeup, like most other luxuries, has served as a tool for separating the elite from lower socioeconomic classes. The Egyptian royalty used kohl (a black powder made up of antimony, or black sulfide). This dark, heavily pigmented makeup greatly increased the contrast of the eyes to the surrounding skin, further highlighting the eyes. In addition to accentuating the eyes, it also served the functional purpose of protecting the eyes from dust and sand.

For a woman, increasing the contrast between light-colored skin and darker eyes further reinforces her femininity.

To test the feminizing benefits of increasing the contrast around the eyes, one study used images of male and female faces that were altered via computer morphing technology (Russell, 2003). The areas around the eyes and mouth

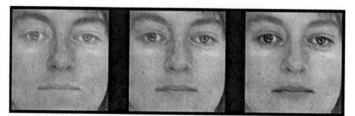

Darkening the eye and mouth areas accentuates the lightness of the surrounding skin and enhances this aspect of feminine beauty. One study used computer morphing technology to show a decreased contrast between the eyes and skin color (left), no change in contrast (center), and increased contrast (right); raters perceived the highest contrast at the right as the most attractive (Russell 2003).

were darkened, but the remainder of the face was left unaltered. Volunteers were then asked to rate the photos on attractiveness, and the results showed a strikingly significant difference between the two sexes. Darkening the eyes and mouth resulted in women being found more attractive; however, when the photos of the males were rated with darkened facial features, they were found to be less attractive. The importance was the contrast between the eyes and the surrounding facial skin.

This study reinforced the impact of one particular signal we subconsciously pick up from facial features. Even though they may have not realized why, men are swept away by women with clear, youthful skin.

Nefertiti and Cleopatra evidently knew that darkened eyes further highlight this femine characteristic. Anything that emphasizes light color and even tones in female facial skin contributes to making a female face appear more beautiful. This is why eye makeup and foundation are the most significant contributors to the enhancement of female attractiveness (Nash et al., 2006). As mentioned earlier, lighter skinned women are better able to abosrb sunlight necessary for manufacturing vitamin D, which is critical for calcium absorbtion—an essential element to prepare the body for pregnancy. It's evolutionarily adaptive for men to be attracted to any physical outward expression of a woman's fertility.

On the other hand, an overly dark appearance around the eyes in men has a negative impact on women. A darkening of the areas around the eyes isn't unusual in men who have a heavy shadowing from a prominent, jutting eyebrow ridge. This is common feature among men with surplus testosterone, and is suggestive of greater dominance. Facial features of excess male dominance signal aggression to the subconscious mind, and alert us to beware. It's not surprising that our most notorious male villains all have darkly contrasted eyes.

Understanding these evolutionary forces makes it easier to understand how makeup came into being as a tool for accentuating femininity and further differentiating themselves from men. Accentuating feminizing traits increases a woman's level of beauty.

Since the eyes are the most important feature of the face for communication and the first place on the face we look, delivering a message of health and beauty starts with accentuating the eyes. The more childlike the eyes, the more attractive a female's face is perceived. Infantile eyes are large; light-colored and slightly further apart than an adult's. A lateral outside corner of the eye that lies just two millimeters slightly above the inside corner of the eye gives an appearance that the eye is slanted upward just ever so slightly, which is considered highly attractive. In addition to this slight slant, eyes that are farther apart have been shown more attractive, regardless of culture (Cunningham et al., 1995). Using makeup to highlight this phenomenon would also be considered attractive, and the beautician that understands the Muller-Lyon optical illusion will know how to use makeup to achieve the most beautiful effect (Fournier, 2002).

Mascara is known to highlight the eyes by increasing the contrast between the eyes and the lids. By extending and darkening the eyelashes, the eyes are framed and highlighted more significantly. Methods to increase the size of the lids include false eyelashes, lash extenders, and the recently FDA-approved Latisse (bimatoprost), an eye-drop drug initially used to treat glaucoma, but also found to grow eyelashes. For years, ophthalmologists noticed that glaucoma patients who used bimatoprost also experienced elongated eyelashes—in fact, they grew to the point that they needed to be trimmed!

The company who makes bimatoprost set up studies with patients to determine if the drug applied directly onto the eyelashes could make the lashes grow. Their studies showed that after 16 weeks of applying the product to the upper eyelashes daily, the lashes were 25% longer, 18% darker, and 106% thicker. The FDA approved the drug

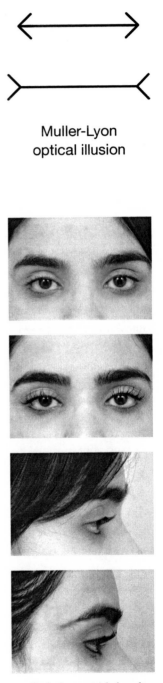

Muller-Lyon optical illusion

Eyelashes extended and thickened with 8 weeks of medical drops

as safe and effective in 2009, and today Latisse is one of the most popular cosmetic drugs on the market. Most women use it daily for about four to five months, and then reduce its use to not overdo it. If they continue to apply it every day, their eyelashes will grow to exorbitant lengths. Side effects have been minimal, from mild irritation to darkening of the eyelids, but once the use is stopped, the eyelashes go back to their normal length. The greatest fear is the theoretical risk of darkening the iris, or the color part of the eye, although as of yet this hasn't been confirmed. In glaucoma patients who get twenty times greater dose of the medicine than a Latisse patient, darkening of the iris has been reported on rare occasions. We can expect this product to remain very popular as it fulfills all the criteria for enhancing the beauty of the eyes.

Trimmed and nicely shaped eyebrows also frame a more attractive appearance to the eyes. We communicate a great deal through the appearance and motions of our eyebrows—slightly elevated eyebrows with a peak just above the outside corner of the eye results in an attractive and friendly impression. Eyebrows that are too bushy are associated with an aged look. Eyebrows that are highly elevated and depressed downward in the midline of the face project an impression of sinister and mean. Too highly elevated eyebrows make someone appear surprised or naïve.

Ideally, the most inviting and youthful-looking eyebrows are appropriately slanted, tweezed, and groomed. When done correctly, waxing and shaping the eyebrows can dramatically improve appearance. Many women who have lost their brows or plucked them excessively use an eyebrow pencil or permanent tattooing to recreate them. But these methods must be very carefully applied, because if the eyebrows appear unnatural, they project a less attractive impression. Not only can the permanent solution of tattooed eyebrows have disastrous cosmetic consequences, they are also very difficult to remove.

> Makeup used to even out and lighten the skin will project an image of youth and virginity.

There are doctors who specialize in transplanting hair to recreate the eyebrow, and while this process can be a very effective permanent solution, it's also pricey. Fortunately, there is growing evidence that Latisse, which I mentioned above, is effective for stimulating eyebrow hair growth as well as lashes. The studies on this use are underway, so stay tuned.

Foundation and Base

In all cultures, females have lighter-colored skin than their male counterparts. The younger a female's age, the fewer dark spots, red blemishes, and the lighter her skin. As stated above, it is widely speculated that lighter-color skin allows a female to absorb more sunlight and, therefore, internally manufacture more vitamin D. Makeup used to homogenize (even out) and lighten the skin will project an image of youth and virginity.

In Asia, as in all cultures, a fair complexion is considered youthful and reinforces images of immaturity, modesty, and lack of expression. Also, in a society where melasma (darkening of the skin) is common, skin lighteners are the most popular of all cosmetics. In Japan, the skin-lightening market is twice the size of America's, despite the fact that the Japanese population is half that of the U.S.

Even in Africa, lighter skin is considered more attractive. Studies that examined the sub-Saharan African cultures found this preference for lighter skin color. These cultures have *not* been exposed to Western media, suggesting that lighter skin is innately considered more attractive in all cultures (Cunningham et al., 1995; van den Berghe & Frost, 1986).

> Making the eyes look bigger deemphasizes the chin, which results in a more feminine-looking face.

Today, we have many prescription and over-the-counter topical creams that bleach the skin. Most are moderately effective, although unable to remove all the dark spots. However, brown discolorations of the face can be greatly reduced with continued use of these creams along with a strong sunscreen.

Makeup foundation and base can also effectively cover up facial discoloration and provide for an even skin tone. Concealer and foundation, along with eye makeup, can be strategically used to make the eyes appear bigger by increasing contrast from the surrounding skin. Making the eyes look bigger deemphasizes the chin, which results in a more feminine-looking face. Women with thicker skin seem to tolerate mineral makeup better than oil-based makeup. Today, many makeup brands include sunscreen that is micronized or compounded directly into the product, which serves the dual purpose of creating a homogenized skin color while simultaneously preventing future sun-initiated blotching of skin.

Tanning

When winter drags on in Chicago, it's hard not to fantasize about sitting on a beach with the sun caressing you from head to toe, followed by a refreshing dip in the infinity pool while sipping a piña colada, the ocean breeze ruffles through your hair. Ahhh . . . but wait! Aren't you forgetting something? Some inner reminder quickly brings you back to reality and veers your thoughts in a new direction—what about the sunscreen?

We've all been flooded with information about the importance of sunscreen and its power to protect from skin damage, premature aging, and skin cancer. Recently I was at a "daddy-daughter" retreat in Mexico with my middle daughter, Alex, and I violated one of the Ten Commandments by forgetting to put on her sunscreen. Oh no! What's going to happen? Is she going to get skin cancer? Age too fast? Maybe she'll melt! What will I tell her mother? What will I tell my mother? But if fairer skin is associated with looking more attractive and youthful, and the dangers of sun exposure are so widely known, why is getting a tan so popular? It's well established that sun exposure is the main cause for the development of skin cancer. Additionally, accelerated skin aging, deeply etched-in wrinkling, and cancerous bodies are directly correlated with too many years of

> Moderate exposure to the sun gives the skin a mild red tone that others subconsciously perceive as being healthy.

sun exposure. With all that in mind, why do we compete to get the best chair on the beach or the patio? Why do rows of people bask in the sun? Is this all just for a sun-kissed look, maybe not. There's a deeper reason we're eager to head out for the rays.

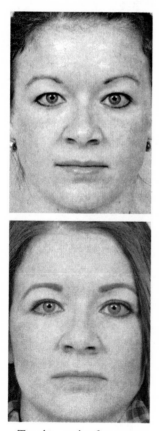

We love the sun, and we love the message hidden in suntanned skin. Moderate sun does make our skin look better in the short-term. The sun causes a slight and temporary thickening and swelling of the skin along with a microscopic enlarging of the blood vessels. The dilated blood vessels transmit a mild reddish hue to the skin, contributing to an appearance that others subconsciously perceive as being healthy. This is one of the reasons for the popularity of blush makeup to highlight the cheeks. Tanning also creates a slight swelling and thickening of the upper layers of the skin, which temporarily reduces the appearance of wrinkles and pore size. The golden brown look also camouflages the aging dark spots that become exposed in the gray, mid-winter months. The result is a more youthful, glowing, and healthier appearance. This perception of tanned skin as more attractive was confirmed in a study in which women were videotaped standing in a neutral pose in their underwear. The videos were shown to both men and women, who rated the attractiveness levels of each subject. The researchers found that tanning was positively correlated with appearing more attractive (Smith, Cornelissen & Tovée, 2007).

Tan skin makes for a more attractive appearance.

Many people turn to sunless tanning products in an attempt to carry a chic, healthy-looking hue while avoiding the damaging effects of the sun. But can a feeling of beauty and bliss really be replicated with a tinting cream? If it were just about looking tan, then a self-tanner should do it, right? Most sunless tanners today use a chemical agent called DHA (dihydroxyacetone) and are safe and effective at achieving a bronzed sheen without the embarrassingly orange shading that used to result from tanners in a tube. However, even with the new sophistication of these products, there's something missing.

The sun's rays seem to directly affect our mood—perhaps the most important reason why many of us adore the sun is that it simply makes us feel better!

It is estimated that one to ten percent of Americans suffer from a form of winter depression known as seasonal affective disorder, or SAD. While it is common for many to develop a mild case of the winter blues, people with SAD can be severely affected to the point that they need medical intervention. Some SAD sufferers even receive light therapy to treat their disease. However, for the majority of us who get a little glum in the winter, a teaspoon of sun might make all the difference in the world. This might be the number one reason we still sit in the sun, regardless of all the warnings and recommendations to the contrary.

Lipstick

Our lips are naturally highlighted with red and pink colors, a sexual trait associated with femininity. Fullest in youth, lips swell ever so slightly during a woman's ovulation and serve as a subconscious signal to men that a woman is fertile. Additionally, a woman's lips may also serve as genital mimickers, appearing to a man's primitive brain like a symbolic indicator of her genitals. A woman's genital lips (labia) will swell and engorge, becoming deeper red

> Makeup applied to improve facial symmetry makes an unattractive face more attractive.

when fertile and ready to mate. The male subconsciously recognizes this as a clue to her fertility and mating status. So, by using lipstick to enlarge, darken, and embolden the lips, a woman sends a man a subconscious clue that she is youthful and fertile.

Creating Symmetry

Makeup is a powerful do-it-yourself tool for enhancing another basic element of beauty— symmetry. We know that a symmetric face subconsciously communicates a message of health and is interpreted as attractive, and from isolated villages in east Africa to the makeup counters of Paris, facial makeup serves the common purpose of making a face appear more symmetric, healthy, and beautiful (Nash et al., 2006). When makeup improves facial symmetry, there is evidence that it makes an unattractive face more attractive (Cárdenas & Harris, 2006). Understanding the value of highlighting feminizing facial features and improving facial symmetry is helpful when learning how to best and most effectively use makeup to communicate a message.

The Clown

While makeup can be used to increase attractiveness, we've all seen women wearing way too much makeup in an attempt to recreate lip lines or eyelids that don't exist, or apply so much foundation that the face appears to be cracking. Is there any chance that this could create a better first impression?

Let's look at the research.

A handful of studies have shown that wearing too much makeup results in projecting a negative impression. The social scientists who have performed these studies have carefully sifted through the results to show that when makeup is inappropriately placed or too heavy, it actually makes a female less attractive (Richetin et al., 2004). This proves the theory that makeup, as well as all cosmetic interventions, have a goal of achieving a natural and subliminal change in one's appearance. If others perceive that too much makeup is being worn, the makeup-plastered woman appears to be hiding or attempting to mask a genetic weakness. This turn-off is nature's way of helping a male avoid wasting his time on a less-than-ideal choice for bearing his future offspring.

> The goal of makeup and other cosmetic interventions is to achieve a natural and subliminal change in one's appearance.

Several studies have shown that applying makeup in a natural and modest way results in feelings of self-confidence and a projected impression of greater self-confidence.

> Unlike women, it's essential for men to avoid increasing the contrast of their facial features, which would make them appear darker and overly aggressive.

Whether wearing makeup promotes an organic increase in self-confidence that is then subtly transferred into a positive alteration in appearance, or the makeup by itself results in a physical improvement in the face perceived by others to be more self-confident, it doesn't really matter. The enhanced projected image of elevated self-esteem, regardless of the mechanism behind it, results in receiving better judgment and treatment from others. Whether preparing for a job interview or social situation, all the evidence shows that it's beneficial to use makeup as a tool to enhance an image. If you're not sure what's best for your distinctive features, you may want to invest in a one-time consult with a professional makeup artist to guarantee that you will bring out your best and, just as important, not overdo it.

Of Makeup and Men

While cosmetic use among men has not been common, it's not entirely uncommon, either. In the past, men primarily used paint for war purposes, but there also have been reports of its use for highlighting facial characteristics. However, unlike women, it's essential

> When the economy goes down, cosmetic sales go up.

for men to avoid increasing the contrast of their facial features, which would make them appear darker and overly aggressive. Traditionally, men have used cosmetic makeup not to masculinize their faces, but rather to hide blemishes and create a healthier, parasite-free image. Yet, men interested in appearing more attractive will gain more benefit from growing out facial hair as a way to highlight their masculine characteristics than from wearing makeup.

However, today there is a "metrosexual" movement that is marked by an increasing awareness and marketing of skin care products for males. Whether or not this trend continues will very much be based on the self-esteem benefits men achieve from such grooming habits.

The Lipstick Effect

Cosmetic sales are less affected by market downturns than other non-essential items, an observation that led to Charles Revson's famously coined term, "the lipstick effect," which refers to the fact that when the economy goes down, lipstick sales go up.

When personal finances are stressed and women look for an affordable, immediately gratifying tool to beautify themselves, facial cosmetics provide an easy answer—regardless of the culture. Estée Lauder, a giant in the field, has been attributed as saying, "After a woman feeds her kids and husband, she will spend money on makeup before feeding herself." The desire to beautify one's self is human nature, and when we think we look good, we feel better. This practice is not unique to Americans. Kalahari bush women use animal fat, even during periods of famine, to moisturize their skin. The ease, safety, and affordability that cosmetics provide for reaching these innate goals indicates that the growth of the cosmetics industry is unlikely to stop anytime soon.

Hair and the First Impression

Many of my family members, including my sister, are deeply religious. They strictly follow the traditions and laws of the Bible and their cultural leaders. One traditional custom in particular is to cover your hair after being married and to comply my sister and cousins when married wear wigs. This custom seems rooted in the need for a taken female to hide a sexually feminizing feature that could attract or express interest to a male suitor. But what's interesting is that my sister and cousins wear expensively designed wigs that in themselves are very attractive. Some of these wigs enhance their facial features even more than their natural

> A better hairstyle can result in ratings of being more caring, warm, sincere, reliable, poised, kind, sensitive, organized, and popular.

hair. But the wigs do prevent them from flipping their hair and using it to diffuse their natural-calling-signal pheromones into the air.

Hair has long had an important impact cosmetically, socially, and functionally. Since the beginning of recorded time, social status and class membership have been represented by hairstyles. In Ancient Egypt, for example, a shaved, bald body except for a lock of hair on the side of the head was a popular symbol of purity for the upper class and was likely a preventative measure against lice. Since the lower socioeconomic classes were more likely to be infested with lice, a hairstyle that could deliver a clear lice-free message to others would send a message that one was disease free and of good gene stock.

The Ancient Greeks also looked to hair to symbolize youth and health. The young commonly have lighter-colored hair, and blonde hair has traditionally had a reputation of being desirable because it symbolizes youth and health. In Ancient Greece, special ointment applied to the hair and then bleached by the sun resulted in blonde hair, which was adored in both men and women. In Asia, depending on the period, long hair often signified nobility and was worn with stunning adornments. In portions of Indian culture, cutting hair is forbidden, and uncut hair is one of the five distinguishing features of Sikhism. In Nigeria, hair braiding dates back to around 500 B.C. and is associated with religion, age, status, and kinship. In Medieval Europe, long, flowing, loose and attractive hair was a mark of an unmarried woman, and to cut it off was a very serious matter. However, married women braided their hair in a tradition that is still seen in many religious and cultural sects in Western and other societies. The Macaroni's, the eighteenth-century suave males from Italy made famous in the "Yankee Doodle Dandy" song for sticking a feather in their caps, wore huge, mountainous wigs of hair to indicate belonging to a group of fashionable young men.

> Brushing our hair gives us confidence and a sense of well-being, order, and control in our appearance.

Today, hairstyles are still used to reveal that one belongs to a certain class of people. From the long hair of a carefree hippie to the crew cuts of the military, a certain hairstyle can be used to send a message. A temporary change in hairstyle can also be effectively used to send a temporary message—a messy hairdo says, "I don't care"; up in a bun states, "I am serious"; and worn long, down, flowing, and wavy says, "I am ready to let loose."

Hairstyles do tell a story, and people do make judgments about one's personality based on their hairstyle. In a study involving models who were evaluated by both unknowing male and female observers before and after hair treatments, it was shown that a better hair style can result in ratings of being more caring, warm, sincere, reliable, poised, kind, sensitive, organized, and popular (Graham & Jouhar, 1981). When you walk into a shop, you likely want to be greeted by someone who appears reliable and kind. This data helps to better understand why some employers and corporations insist on a certain hairstyle.

Most people brush their hair just prior to leaving the house. It's as much a habit as brushing our teeth. Why is it so second nature?

Brushing hair is more than just grooming—it provides us with confidence and a sense of well-being, order, and control in our appearance. Many social scientists and clinicians have reported the self-esteem-boosting benefits of getting our hair done (Getz & Klein, 1980; Patzer). From all walks of life, and from depressed patients to the elderly, getting a hairdo not only results in making a better impression, but also in feeling better about oneself.

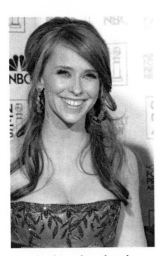

Big hair dimishes the appearance of the chin.

Hairstyles and their uses are rooted in their functional ability to increase attractiveness. The youth tend to have thick, colorful hair with a lot of body to it, whereas the elderly have hair that is thin, fragile, and gray. Hair also can provide valuable information about one's health. Since the hair at the end of your head has been there for many months, it can reveal information about the metabolic processes of your body at the time it was created. However, those who suffer from chronic diseases may lose their hair or have hair color changes. This serves as a clue to others that one's genes may be less than optimal. Long, thick hair is associated with feminine youth, and men prefer long hair and other signs of youthfulness. And long hair, as mentioned previously, is also found by many men to be very sexually appealing because they can unconsciously pick up the pheromones released when a woman flips her hair. Because apocrine glands and pheromone secreting glands can be found in the scalp, the long hair is a way to send a scent further into the environment and let the potential mate know that a female is interested (Grammer et al., 2003).

This helps explain why certain cultures forbid married woman to expose their hair. The sexual calling properties of hair affect our subconscious minds, and covering women's hair prevents those signals from spreading through the air. However, in some cultures women choose to not expose their hair as a way of telling others they are off the market and not interested. Whether or not this is actually how they feel is another thing, but that is the cultural purpose of the covering. Women can't control sending out chemical signals about their heightened fertility, and covering the hair is one way to prevent any confusion.

The rarer the hair color in a population, the more likely the genes within that person are more diverse and therefore a better match to produce a more fit offspring.

Plentiful hair can strategically be used to improve appearance in many ways, such as wearing bangs to cover up a high hairline that would otherwise expose the forehead and make a woman look older. While the big hairstyles of the eighties may not be considered fashionable today, they were certainly valuable to those women with a large chin and lower one-third of their faces. A prominent chin and jawline are male characteristic traits that women try to diminish in order to create a more attractive appearance. Big hair tends to take the emphasis away from the lower third and can be an advantage in providing a more feminine appearance.

Rare Hair

We've seen that lighter-colored hair is considered attractive because of its association with youth. We're also drawn to a rare color, because the rarer the hair color in a population, the more likely the genes within that person are more diverse and therefore a better match to produce a more fit offspring (Grammer et al., 2003).

As a female ages, her hair darkens. Is this why men prefer blondes? And why the majority of models in U.S. magazines are blonde?

In a study we performed in 2009, we asked our female patients if they dyed their hair, and if so, what color (Dayan, Arkins & Mussman, 2011). Seventy percent of our sample patients reported that they dyed their hair, and blonde was the most popular color. The most common natural hair color of a patient was brunette

> Men like what they are not used to—some prefer blondes, and other brunettes.

(sixty-one percent). For patients who dyed their hair, they maintained this color for an average of thirteen years with forty-five percent maintaining the color for more than ten years. Beyond finding that more women prefer to dye their hair blonde, we confirmed that women are more open about changing their hair color. What was secret and taboo in the 1950s is now common and ordinary.

If women seem to prefer going blonde, the next questions are obvious: do blondes really have more fun? Do they appeal more to men?

The answer may surprise you.

> Men with a regular quantity of hair are rated as most handsome, virile, and sharp, while balding men are rated least potent, weak, dull, and inactive.

Men describe blondes as beautiful, rich, and feminine and brunettes as intelligent and familiar, but they seem to vary on which they prefer (Synnott, 1987). In an evaluation of men's preferences, it turns out that men like what they are not used to, and this would make evolutionary sense because the hair color you are not used to would indicate a different gene pool. This would be more desirable, because it means mating with someone whose genes are more different from your own and increasing the chance of having a fit offspring. So, some prefer blondes, and others brunettes (Synnott, 1987; Thelen, 1983). In either case, grey hair is associated with aging, and is one of the primary signs that tips us off that someone is aging or older (Gunn et al., 2009).

Men's Hair

Many men are incredibly concerned with their hair. Their self-esteem goes up or down depending on their hair loss or graying. Gray hair signifies age and a lowered ability to provide for offspring. However, a small amount of gray may be associated with resourcefulness, because in today's culture, men in their thirties to early fifties are more likely to have accumulated resources.

There are a few important issues to keep in mind if a man is thinking about dying his hair. If he wants to look more youthful, coloring out the gray will have that effect. What about going lighter? Blonde hair, as we've seen, is associated with youth and can be perceived as attractive, but those who lack pigmentation and have almost white hair are typically not considered attractive. Likewise, redheads tend to have features not found attractive. In fact, in one survey women described male redheads as good, but effeminate, timid, and weak (Horn, 1979). For redheaded men, dyeing their hair a bit darker may make sense.

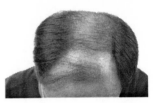

Combover draws attention to a baliding head

And while male pattern balding, or androgenic alopecia, is common in Western society, many men still try to fight the loss. From over-the-counter lotions and hair weaves to medical and surgical options, there is no shortage of attempts to find the cure for baldness. Today's $600 million market for treating baldness in the U.S. reflects how strongly men correlate their hair with their self-esteem. A full head of hair is a strong indicator of a man's vitality. We all know what happened to Samson when he lost his hair, and, as painful as it may sound to hair-challenged men, studies prove that men with a regular quantity of hair are rated as most handsome, virile, strong, active, and sharp, and the balding male is rated least potent, weak, dull, inactive, more unkind, and ugly (Roll & Verinis, 1971).

Full head of hair is associated with youth, and up until their forties, men with more hair are found to be more attractive and youthful. Furthermore, we like our leaders to have a full head of hair. Of our forty-three presidents, twenty-five percent were balding, whereas in the general population the number is fifty percent. The same goes with U.S. senators.

Fixing Hair Loss

Great hair definitely has its advantages, and men and women will be relieved to learn that there are many preventive remedies and treatments for hair loss. The first such drug produced for this condition was Minoxidil, which was originally developed in the 1970s to treat high blood pressure. Men and women treated with the drug noted hair growth on their faces and head. This led to studies with Minoxidil placed topically onto the head. In 1988, Minoxidil became the first FDA-approved drug for hair loss, and in 1996 it was approved as an over-the-counter version. While Minoxidil does seem to provide many men and women with a reduction in hair loss, only about thirty percent of men can expect to see cosmetically significant results. Even more disappointing, in some men, the side effects of dropping their blood pressure can become intolerable.

> Today's more natural-looking hair implants can deliver a life-changing jolt of confidence.

The second FDA-approved drug for hair loss came along in 1998 under similar circumstances. When it first came on the market in the early 1990s, the popular medication Proscar (finasteride) prescribed for men with enlarged prostate also produced an unusual ability to prevent hair loss and cause the growth of new hair. The prostate gland, a secretory gland at the base between the bladder and the penis, envelops the urethra, the conduit through which urine and semen exits the penis and contributes fluid to semen. As men age, the prostate gland enlarges and can cause obstruction of the urine, and many also develop prostate cancer with age. Proscar has been shown to reduce the size of the prostate, and the serendipitous side effect of hair growth led to studies using a lower dose of the medication. The rather remarkable results showed statistically significant regrowth of hair in over ninety percent of men between the ages of eighteen and forty-one.

However, once men stop taking the drug, the gains reverse and controversy surrounds whether or not it decreases libido and causes erectile dysfunction and depression. These reactions were noted in up to four percent of patients. While this drug seems to be very beneficial for maintaining and growing hair, it also has proven important to prostate health resulting in many doctors recommending taking it every day. This drug is not safe in women who are pregnant and its safety and effectiveness has yet to be proven in post-menopausal women.

> Like too much makeup on a woman, ineffective attempts to hide balding hair indicate to the subconscious mind of the unknowing observer that the man is hiding a genetic weakness.

Recent studies with light-based devices, or "lasers," to grow hair have been met with mixed results. The emitted light is thought to stimulate the metabolic process of the hair cell to induce growth of the hair. This makes sense in theory, especially for those with just thinning hair that have not yet permanently lost hair. In 2008, we did a study with an FDA-approved device for thinning hair in women, and our findings were not impressive. Despite its popularity, it is hard to recommend this treatment.

Surgical solutions are the most permanent solution for hair loss, and include hair transplants, where single, double and triple hairs are taken from denser areas at the back of the head and reinserted to the front and top balding areas of the head. While early results with this technique often left many men appearing very unnatural and doll-like, today the results are very natural when done by an experienced hair transplant surgeon. Men with lighter, curlier hair seem to do better, but great results can be seen in all hair colors, ethnicities, and in both genders. I've seen many men and women who have undergone transplants, and it can deliver a life-changing jolt of confidence.

Non-surgical options for hair loss include toupees, hair weaves, and wigs. This is nothing new, of course—seventeenth-century gentlemen famously wore wigs because it was an easy way to hide evidence of balding. However, many men today don't like the feeling or necessary upkeep of wearing a wig. And traditionally, hair wigs for men have been very obvious. From Howard Cosell to Sam Donaldson and others, bad toupees can look garishly unnatural and be a real detriment to one's appearance. Regardless of the method of attempting to hide the baldness, whether a bad wig, noticeable hair plugs, or a comb-over, all these methods actually have the opposite effect. Just like too much makeup on a woman, they indicate to the subconscious mind of the unknowing observer that the man is hiding a genetic weakness (Grammer et al., 2003). Therefore, men who are balding and considering treatment options, whether a toupee, hair weave, or hair transplant surgery, it is absolutely critical that it be done well.

Today, hair transplants are one of the most popular cosmetic procedures for males. In some cases, when one is not a good candidate for surgery or a toupee, it may be best to shave the head completely bald. Michael Jordan, Dwayne "The Rock" Johnson, Vin Diesel, and Jason Statham are all considered male sex symbols, and all have little to no visible hair on their heads. Remember, the human eye looks for contrast, and a receding hairline or a bad camouflaging attempt is consistent with aging.

Latisse (bimatoprost), the drug mentioned above for eyelash growth, is stirring up a lot of excitement because it may be an effective treatment for baldness. The enormous financial potential of finding a drug to cure baldness has prompted trials evaluating its safety and effectiveness. With so much at stake, early reports are being held top secret. If this drug proves successful at curing baldness—wow! Both men and women would have an option for greatly enhancing one of the most vital signs of attractiveness.

CHAPTER 10

SLEEP LIKE A BABY, EAT LIKE A CAVEMAN

"Sometimes we get caught up in what we need to do next and forget about what are the very essential and important things in life. I treasure my time to sleep. It's just as important as eating or exercise."

—Jennifer Lopez

Three lifestyle basics—adequate sleep, good nutrition, and moderate exercise—are as essential to feeling and looking better as the confidence-boosting techniques already discussed. Unfortunately, the first thing we seem to toss aside in our busy lives is taking care of ourselves. Although the hardest part about shifting into a healthier lifestyle is actually getting started, if we're really interested in making a better first impression, there's no substitute for giving our bodies the rest, nutrition and healthy activity that is needed.

Beauty Sleep Is No Myth

According to the National Commission on Sleep Disorder Research, sleepiness can become so problematic that it can disrupt our daily activities, and between .05 and 5 percent of the population suffer from problem due to lack of sleep. "Moreover," says this group, "it is not clear that persons with excessive sleepiness fully appreciate the problems it poses" (National Center on Sleep Disorders Research and Office of Prevention, 1977).

Over the last hundred years, cultural and economic forces have cut our average amount of nightly sleep by more than twenty percent.

Problem sleepiness in the United States is more likely to be due to lifestyle factors than to specific sleep disorders. Over the last hundred years, cultural and economic forces have cut our average amount of nightly sleep by more than *twenty percent* (Roth, 1995).

The exact function of sleep remains a mystery, but we know that one-third of our life is necessarily spent sleeping, and it appears that many important physiological functions take place during those hours. Everyone requires a different amount of sleep. Some people are replenished with as little as five hours, while others need ten hours, but most people require about seven-and-a-half to eight-and-a-half hours of sleep every night. As we age, we lose some of our ability to enter deep and restorative sleep, and women may be affected the same way during premenstrual periods and menopause. Anxiety, alcohol,

Not getting enough sleep decreases the function of our immune system and makes us more prone to gaining weight.

and a variety of medical conditions affect sleep patterns as well. However, most sleep difficulties relate to lifestyle choices—which we can completely control.

When we don't make it a priority to get enough sleep, we compromise every aspect of our health. The effects of sleep deprivation are significant, including increasing fatigue, a decrease in cognitive skills, and mood imbalances. Those who are sleep deprived may have a decrease in immune system function, release less growth hormone, and are more prone to weight gain (Evans, Kennedy & Wertheim, 2005; Patel, Malhotra, White, Gottlieb & Hu, 2006). Sleep deprivation is also linked to increased heart rate variability (Ewing, Neilson, Shapiro, Stewart & Reid, 1991).

Clearly, the amount of sleep we get affects our mood, but does the quantity of sleep directly affect our appearance? What exactly does that mean—to look tired? A 2010 study done in Stockholm attempted to define if tired people look different (Axelsson et al., 2010).

They recruited volunteers who were photographed after a normal night of sleep and then again after a night of limited sleep, around five hours, those who had only five hours of sleep were noted to appear on average less healthy, less attractive, and more tired.

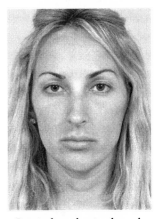

Being sleep deprived can be detected in appearance.

As the researcher Axelsson wrote, "Sleep-deprived people appear less healthy, less attractive and more tired compared with when they are well rested. Humans are sensitive to sleep-related facial cues." So, yes, it does appear that others can detect when someone has been sleep deprived.

Sleep is important to how you feel and ultimately how you look. The appearance of sleep deprivation, no matter how natural or self-inflicted, can lead to projecting a subliminal message that you are in poor health.

Chocolate Good, Sugar Bad

There's no doubt that American eating habits are not healthy. Obesity in the U.S. is epidemic, and our children are headed to disaster. As of 2012, 17 percent of our children and adolescents are obese, three times the amount of a generation ago (Centers for Disease Control and Prevention, 2012). According to Nielsen, Americans purchase around fifty-eight million pounds of chocolate during the days leading up to Valentine's Day. The sweetheart holiday only surpassed by Halloween, when we buy about 598 million pounds or $1.9 billion worth of candy, of which nearly ninety million pounds is chocolate!

> The ups and downs of blood sugar levels that come from eating excessive sugar leads to inflammation, the foundation of many diseases, and makes us feel bloated and sluggish.

We've looked at why sugar is sweet and why we like it, but what about chocolate? Why do we crave it so much? Like sugar, the desirable taste of chocolate is not coincidental. Moderate amounts of dark chocolate are high in antioxidants and its health benefits range from lowering blood pressure and bad cholesterol to reducing dementia. While sugary fruit gave our prehistoric ancestors a quick energy boost, we also evolved an irresistible attraction to beans from the cocoa plant to ensure that we would gain from its benefits. Chocolate lovers will be happy to learn that about 3.5 ounces of dark chocolate a day is good for your heart. Eating more than that, however, adds too many calories to your diet, so, like sugar, dark chocolate should be eaten in small amounts.

Foods with high sugar content such as sodas, sweetened breads, and candy bars are known to raise blood sugars rapidly, resulting in a quick energy spike followed by a big drop in blood sugar, which result in tiredness and hunger again. This cycle is not healthy, as it leads to long-term inflammation and injury to cells. Over time, excess sugar in the body can negatively affect many organs, including the largest organ, the skin. This

> The longest lifespans in the world are found on the Japanese island of Okinawa, where people consume a diet high in fish and leafy green vegetables and low in complex carbohydrates and sugar.

accelerates the aging appearance of the skin. Excess sugar in the diet is speculated to affect collagen fibers, resulting in a process called glycation that can result in a yellow color to the skin

While it makes sense that a diet high in sugars is not ideal for the skin, it's also easy to see how dramatically it can alter the way you feel. The ups and downs in sugar levels makes you feel stuffed or bloated and, ultimately, the weight gain can lead to a sluggish disposition.

The Popeye Effect

When I was a kid, I never stopped being amazed at how Popeye sprouted instant muscles and saved the day after guzzling down a can of spinach. I asked for spinach and swallowed it down whole while pinching my nose. Spinach doesn't give us immediate supernatural energy, of course, but the popular cartoon may have been on to something. Spinach is chock full of nutrients including powerful antioxidants, anti-inflammatories, and cancer-fighting flavonoids. And one cup of spinach contains three times the recommended daily allowance of Vitamin A, an essential element for skin health.

But for those who aren't fans of spinach and are set on actively doing all they can to make their skin look its best, supplemental nutritional products can work wonders. Multiple quality studies have shown the health-protecting benefits of antioxidants as part of a healthy diet. In fact, it's no coincidence that the longest lifespans in the world are found on the Japanese island of Okinawa, where people consume a diet high in fish and leafy green vegetables and low in complex carbohydrates and sugar. Multiple studies have also detailed the benefits that antioxidants, either taken as a pill or placed on the skin, can have against the DNA-damaging ultraviolet rays of the sun (Cesarini, Michel, Maurette, Adhoute & Bejot, 2003; Darr, Combs, Dunston, Manning & Pinnell, 1992; Darr, Dunston, Faust & Pinnell, 1996; Diffey, 2002; Gensler & Magdaleno, 1991; Ryan & Goldsmith, 1996).

The best known of the antioxidants for helping fight heart disease and inflammation is vitamin E, which is also an important skin protector. Vitamin E wards off and reverses damage inflicted on the skin from too much sun or other insults that can lead to rapid skin aging. By increasing the vitamin E levels in the skin, it appears that the tissue will not sustain as much damage, repair injured cells faster, and improve its overall appearance. Researchers have found that taking 400 IU vitamin E pills orally will increase the concentration of vitamin E in the skin

> Vitamin E is the best-known antioxidant for fighting heart disease and inflammation.

(McArdle et al., 2004). This higher concentration provides added protection against sun damage and aging skin. However, it takes two to three weeks of supplementation for enough vitamin E to build up to start its age-combating benefits.

Vitamin C is also a potent antioxidant that enhances the skin by helping with collagen synthesis and wound healing. However, taking additional oral ingestion of vitamin C doesn't seem to have much of a direct effect on reversing the appearance of fine lines and wrinkles. Other nutritional supplements such as lycopene, coenzyme-Q10, minerals such as zinc, and botanicals such as green tea all may be beneficial to the appearance of the skin by reducing inflammation.

While the evidence is mounting that supplementation is good for you, we just don't know for sure how much and what amount to take. The variation within the many different products makes it difficult for physicians to know which brand of supplement to recommend. In a current health environment where sixty percent of Americans are now seeking alternative care options outside of traditional medicine, clinical trials aimed at a better understanding of the risks, benefits, and limitations of nutritional supplements is not only necessary, but should become mandatory.

In 2011, we published data on a clinical trial evaluating the benefits of an oral nutritional supplement manufactured by Standard Process Inc. Palmyra Wisconsin called SHEP (Skin Health Experimental Product) on skin (Dayan & Arkins, 2011). This nutritional supplement pill is comprised of natural, whole food-based elements including but not limited to omega-3 fatty acids, ascorbic acid, beta-carotene, zinc, pyridoxine, niacin, and coenzyme-Q10. Among the more than 100 men and women enrolled into our study, half took the SHEP product twice a day for nine months and the other half took a placebo pill (pill with no antioxidants). Throughout the trial, we evaluated the depth of facial skin wrinkles around the eyelid skin, antioxidant levels in the skin, skin hydration levels, and facial appearance to unknowing judges. We also asked the patients in the study to self-rate how they looked.

> People who took the oral nutritional supplement in our study had fewer wrinkles, higher antioxidant levels in their skin, and reported that they felt they looked better.

We found that those who took the supplement had significant reduction in fine-line facial wrinkles, increased antioxidant levels in the skin, and also felt they looked better. This was one of the first well-designed studies on nutritional supplements, and we concluded that it provided new evidence to support that oral nutritional supplementation can improve the way one appears, even though the improvement is subtle. What impressed me even more was the statistically significant difference in how those who took SHEP believed they looked. Their positive experience indicated to me that the products might make people feel better about their own appearance, and I'm convinced that one's self-esteem is the most essential component of looking better. As a result, in my office we now offer nutritional supplements to all our patients, especially those that are undergoing surgery. We want to do our best to optimize their care and outcomes.

If you would like to add nutritional supplements to your health regimen, I suggest you meet with a physician knowledgeable in this area for a complete physical exam, nutritional evaluation, and up-to-date information rather than just going to the nutrition store and buying whatever is on the shelf. Keep in mind, not all the nutritional supplements that are purchased over-the-counter are similar. They are manufactured very differently and aren't regulated by the Food and Drug Administration to the same extent as drugs—they have to prove that they are safe but not that they work. I believe that over the next decade, nutrition will become an increasingly important ingredient in preventing and treating disease and a major component for looking your best. Moreover, even if a nutritional supplement does not directly affect the skin, changing lifestyle and eating habits improves your mood and ultimately leads to making a better first impression.

Keep It Movin'

When our middle daughter, Alex, was sick and we spent many days in and out of the hospital, the days were long and the evenings even longer. It was a difficult time for me and my wife. Our hearts and minds were heavy with worry and stress, but we both found enormous solace in running.

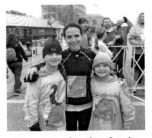

Elise, my wife, after finishing a marathon with my two daughters who ran the 5K and met her at the end.

We took breaks at the hospital and swapped responsibilities so one of us could go for a run along the Chicago lakefront. This always seemed to clear the mind and refill our tolerance reservoir for another stint of stress. It's not surprising to learn that running releases brain chemicals called endorphins that help elevate our mood. Running is a natural way to feel good. My wife was able to train and complete a marathon during this time period. Fortunately, today our daughter is a healthy and rambunctious eleven year old and running continues to be a normal regimen for both of us.

According to one physician and writer, physical fitness is the magic bullet when it comes to our health and by just taking two ten-minute walks a day we can decrease our "real age" by nearly two years.

Those who exercise regularly seem to be healthier in both appearance and mood. While there is little doubt that exercise brings physical benefits, it's now well accepted that regular exercise can also lead to significant improvements in cognitive function and mood (Hendricks, McEwen & Ouderaa, 2005). Humans were designed to run in the plains and jungles, work the fields, and till the crops. We were not constructed to sit in a chair or couch all day in poorly ventilated rooms. Moderate exercise helps the brain release many beneficial chemicals that elevate mood and also improve the ability for cells to take up oxygen and use nutrients. Exercise decreases blood pressure, reduces bad cholesterol, increases good cholesterol, and improves our ability to manage blood sugar levels and our chances for living a longer life. Incorporating an exercise regimen will change the way you look physically rather quickly. Exercise improves vascularity, which gives a homogenous (uniform), pinkish healthy hue to facial skin that is subconsciously perceived by others as healthy, youthful, and attractive (Johnson, 1998; Stephen, Coetzee, Law Smith & Perrett, 2009). In a European study published in 2009, participants were allowed to adjust the facial color on faces until they appeared most healthy (Stephen et al., 2009). The researchers found that a homogenous or an unbroken up diffuse redness to the skin was associated with a healthier appearance. This finding is consistent with many other studies that have revealed that faces with a reddish hue are more attractive.

> Exercise doesn't have to be a Herculean effort in order to give us benefits.

What's so attractive about a pinkish flush?

This coloring is associated with better oxygenation and vascularity of the skin. When it's not apparent, such as in the discolored or pale skin of those with cardiovascular disease, anemia, diabetes, or jaundice, we perceive this coloring as a lack of health. Evolutionary directives have guided our subconscious minds to identify an even pink/reddish tint on facial skin as healthy and thereby attractive. Moderate, regular exercise is an all-natural way to create this healthy glow.

In addition to physically helping us project a more attractive appearance, moderate exercise also promotes self-esteem, confidence, and an elevated mood (McAuley, Mihalko & Bane, 1997). In a Psychology Today survey, exercise ranked as an important self-enhancing action we can take to improve health, mood and the way we feel about our appearance. Because elevated self-esteem is the most important aspect of projecting a more favorable first impression, exercise is a great way to move closer to that goal. Exercise doesn't have to be a Herculean effort in order to give us benefits, but please check with your physician prior to beginning an exercise routine.

> Men are not programmed to desire a wafer-thin, unhealthy-looking woman.

Some Americans are motivated to go beyond the health benefits of routine exercise and are adopting extensive strength training programs designed to bulk-up with muscle. Others push aerobic exercise and calorie restriction to the limit in an effort to trim down to a wafer-thin body. Some athletes, models, and even regular folks use illegal supplements such as androgenic anabolic steroids, usually in the form of a male hormone, to reach these goals. While they can help create bulky muscles and a very tight and trim midsection, such methods come at a price. The negative effects go beyond the pain of the steroid injection. Higher levels of male hormones result in acne, shrunken testes, mood rages, short stature, and an increased risk for cancer, heart disease, and even death. Women who take steroids to help build a strong physique may start to grow facial and body hair and will stop menstruating. And while it's important for parents to keep their kids away from these substances, which are now readily available at some high schools, adults can make up their own minds about the risks.

But are the extremes worth it?

Does anyone find these overly buff or rail-thin figures attractive? We know from biological studies that our primitive female ancestors were attracted to men with resourcefulness, which came in the form of large pectoral muscles and big shoulders that could be used to fend off threats or capture dinner. But as detailed in Chapter four, hyper-masculine males characterized by low set brows, overly prominent chins, low hairlines, and overly bulging muscles are considered threatening rather than attractive by many women. Men, on the other hand, are attracted to an hourglass figure with supple curves because this is a sign of a healthy, fertile female. They're not programmed to desire a wafer-thin, unhealthy-looking woman. Therefore, it seems that massive amounts of exercise, illegal substances, and excessive caloric restriction can lead to a less-than-ideal figure.

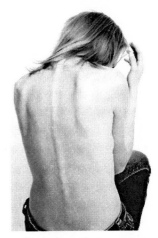

Anorexic patient, a serious medical condition

Regardless of how much we exercise, however, not everyone can have ideal hour-glass figures like Heidi Klum, Jennifer Lopez, and Salma Hayek, or hunky physiques and masculine features like Ryan Reynolds, Jason Statham, and Brad Pitt. We are all made differently and should celebrate and work with what we've got. It's true, however, that feeling positive about one's beauty is neither simple nor common for many women around the world, and it's a lifelong process that starts early in life.

> Nine out of ten women want to change something about their appearance—most commonly their body weight and shape.

In a large, multicultural study with women from six continents, seven out of ten reported that they refrained from daily activities when they didn't feel good about themselves (Etcoff et al., 2006). So much of how a young female gains self-esteem and self-worth is rooted within the mother-daughter relationship. There is evidence that the ideas and behaviors of mothers start to influence a daughter's body image during their first years of life, resulting in nine out of ten women wanting to change something about their appearance—most commonly their body weight and shape.

Regardless of where the influence comes from, we are witnessing an epidemic of teenagers and young adults who do not accurately see themselves. They may suffer from a medical disease known as body dysmorphic disorder (BDD), which affects one percent of the U.S. population. Sufferers of this condition, which affects both men and women and is more common in adolescents, become preoccupied with a body part or its influence on their overall appearance. The most common physical features for a BDD person to focus in on are body weight, skin and the nose. In fact it is estimated that somewhere between 3 to 15% of patients seeking a nasal reshaping procedure (rhinoplasty) may be affected by BDD. Regardless of the body feature, these patients constantly need to check themselves in a mirror, may think that others are staring at them, and often lack self-confidence. Some eventually drop all social contact and become homebound.

In a related condition, young girls who strive for a look that may not be natural and certainly not healthy, restrict calories and essentially starve themselves or binge and purge in attempt to gain a thin appearance. This is commonly referred to as anorexia nervosa, and when severe, the body starts to digest itself. These victims only see themselves as fat, despite being skin and bones. Death is a real possibility for anorexics, and is the ultimate course for ten percent of those diagnosed (Birmingham, Su, Hlynsky, Goldner & Gao, 2005). While females from wealthy, white families seem to be most affected (Lindberg & Hjern, 2003), men are increasingly being recognized as suffering from this condition.

All of our health-enhancing lifestyle changes, from diet to exercise, should be done in moderation. Exercising is a lifelong habit that needs to become a routine part of existence and not a chore to struggle through. To enjoy and stay with a habit of exercise, consider something that's also fun. For example, play basketball with friends, go on long walks with a loved one, garden, swim, or do yoga or Pilates with your girlfriends. All of these work to strengthen your muscles and help clear your mind. There are so many ways to incorporate exercise into our daily routines that can be fun and worthwhile rather than a burden.

> To become part of your life, exercise should be fun: play basketball with friends, garden, walk with a loved one, or do yoga with your girlfriends.

Projecting a favorable impression requires the natural elements of adequate sleep, proper nutrition, and moderate exercise. Each is basic to any healthy lifestyle, but unfortunately, many do not get enough of these essentials in the appropriate doses. As we get older, youth-defining normal hormone levels such as testosterone and estrogen grow and drop respectively, leading to disrupted sleep cycles, fatigue, mood disorders, and a reduction in cognitive skills. We can't avoid the fundamental hormonal changes of aging, but we can choose to take a new look at our priorities.

Today, there is a movement called Age Management Medicine, or Anti-Aging Medicine which we can expect to become very popular and mainstream in the near future.

Doctors who are proponents of this movement argue that the goal is to not make you live longer, but healthier. When I was in medical school, this was considered heretical and fringe thinking. We were taught that eating a balanced meal would provide all the necessary vitamins and minerals we needed, and ideas about antioxidants and fish oil supplements were considered radical. These concepts are now readily accepted.

> The goal of Age Management Medicine is not to make you live longer, but healthier.

Pioneering doctors recommend taking a preventative instead of reactive approach to disease. In other words, medicine should be about optimizing our health so that we are less susceptible to the illnesses and diseases associated with aging in the first place.

There is good science to show that by getting adequate sleep, exercising, eating right, and restricting our diets from carbohydrates and sugars, we can feel better, prevent disease, and look better. Adequate sleep results in energy reserves, making the rhythmic cycles of the day so much easier to manage. Moderate exercise, that at first may seem burdensome, soon starts to be a means to a natural and enjoyable high. And once you reduce your intake of high sugar foods, you begin to lose your cravings.

The consistent mood elevation that comes from all of these positive changes will make others begin to notice a healthier and more youthful appearance. The key is to act with moderation and in the case of eating right, to never say the word "diet." Once declared that you're restricting yourself, you've lost. Every part of this regimen only works when it becomes a regular and enjoyable part of a lifestyle.

Even though we live in very different environments than our primitive ancestors, with our own stresses and priorities, we would do well to follow their example. Good sleep, natural food, and regular exercise molded us into the extraordinary species we are today—smart, strong and ready for anything. To fulfill our greatest potential physically, mentally, and emotionally, we should listen to our inner caveman or woman, who tells us to get a full night's sleep, eat food straight from Mother Nature, and get off our behinds and go for a walk.

CHAPTER 11

PRIMAL MEDICINE

"A very subtle difference can make the picture or not."
—Annie Leibovitz

The Unified Theory of Beauty

Early in my career I saw a sixty-eight-year-old lady in consultation who had a heavy face, sagging neck skin, puffy eyes, and deep wrinkles. When I first met her, she was shy and hesitant to tell me her concerns, but after a few minutes of chatting and learning more about her, she opened up and told me that what she really desired was a smaller and cuter nose.

"OK," I said. "What bothers you about it?" I was surprised that this was her major concern. While her nose was slightly enlarged and droopy, it was not the area on her face that most detracted from a youthful or more attractive appearance. Upon further discussion, she revealed to me that her husband of fifty years and former high school sweetheart had just passed away. And since her grammar school days, when kids had always teased her about her nose, she had always dreamed of having her nose "fixed," but her husband was against the surgery. Now that he had passed on, she was going to go ahead and have it done. It was very interesting to learn that she was still so hurt by the teasing after all these years. The childish ridicule that she received at an early age imprinted into her personality and deep down she still saw herself as the ostracized little girl. She wasn't at all bothered by other signs of aging on her face. So I reduced the size of her nose and she was pleased, and to this day every year during the holidays she sends our office a large gift basket.

Another patient came to me with a similar intent. I participate in a program called Face to Face, which runs through my Facial Plastic Surgery Academic Society (AAFPRS) and offers treatment at no cost to victims of domestic violence. A curse on society, domestic violence is the leading cause of injury to women—more than car accidents, muggings, and rapes combined. Unfortunately, many of these women are afraid to leave their situations and succumb to further abuse. In 2008, I saw a thirty-five-year-old lady who came in on this program complaining of a horrendous scar on her left cheek. When I met her, I couldn't see the mark. She kept pointing to the same spot, insisting it was disfiguring and saying, "Can't you see it? Look closer!"

I put on magnifying glasses and could then see a small, round mark that had a slightly depressed inner core. She told me it was the scar from where her ex-husband hit her with a key, and its appearance really bothered her. "What can you do to get rid of it?" she asked. It was obvious that this scar, which the naked eye could barely detect, didn't capture anyone's attention, but that didn't matter. To her the scarring ran much deeper, touching her innermost fears. It was a scar of the heart and a constant reminder of what she had been through. And now that she had the courage to leave her husband and was moving on with her life, she needed this memento lifted. I did a minor laser resurfacing procedure, further camouflaging the scar's appearance, and while the improvement I created was slight and wouldn't be noticed by the unknowing observer, it made a significant impact on her life and well-being. In reality, I was treating so much more than a facial scar. And she was much better off for it. She was instantly happier, became an ambassador for the program, and went on to a new chapter in her life.

> In 2010, there were over nine million cosmetic procedures performed in the United States, and most of them were non-surgical.

We each may have a specific reason for wanting something altered. Many people seek out a cosmetic surgeon to regain the youthful appearance they once cherished or enhance a sexual characterizing trait. Sometimes the desire stems from a need to alleviate a reminder of a physical or social trauma. The valuable lesson for me gained from both of these women is that what bothers each of us about our appearance may have nothing to do with whether or not it's obvious to others.

In 2010, there were over nine million cosmetic procedures performed in the United States, and most of them were non-surgical treatments. For some, cosmetic reconstructive surgery can be a miraculous endeavor, allowing a disfigured victim the ability to regain self-esteem and reentry back into society. For those with a disproportioned nose that deviates from an otherwise very balanced face, rhinoplasty, or nose reshaping, can allow the patient's more attractive facial features to become prominent. I have always been convinced that other, less obvious and more important positive effects of plastic surgery that can impact people's lives are being glossed over by both doctors and conventional wisdom. Otoplasty, or ear pinning surgery, may prevent a lifetime of emotional scarring for a first grader who the kids call Dumbo. Others, like my hairdresser friend whose appearance makes people misjudge him as mean, feel that wrinkle-reducing filler treatments are a must-have for their livelihoods. Contrary to the stereotypes, most people seeking out cosmetic procedures are not rich, vain, or self-centered. In a 2011 study, we showed that people getting Botox are no more concerned with their appearance than those coloring their hair. Plastic surgery is moving far beyond altering a nose, lips, or chin. Something deeper, more impacting, and substantial is motivating people to make changes. What brought about this increasing acceptance? To answer that, let's take a look at the origins of plastic surgery and see how it's evolved.

An Ancient Art

From the de-branding of slaves to the reversal of disfiguring scars on ancient warriors, I believe that improving one's self-esteem has long been the goal of cosmetic surgery. Plastic surgery has its roots in the Greek and Roman empires, in which conquered nomadic populations attempting to integrate into these societies wanted to hide body-marking evidence of a nefarious past or belonging to an unacceptable cult. Rather than treatments for enhancing the beauty of the elite, these early procedures were more of a service trade allowing disenfranchised people to pass into society or blend in without being noticed or discriminated. In a society where nudity was celebrated, the first cosmetic surgeries were performed on early Hebrews and Druze who desired circumcision reversal. Likewise, to merge into society unnoticeably, scars on the back were often a sign of losing in battle or being a previous slave, and these individuals wanted to reverse distinguishing marks. Cosmetic medicine wasn't limited to the ancient Europeans. Ancient Indian doctors created methods for replacing the noses of warriors who had had them ceremonially amputated following a loss in battle.

Modern cosmetic surgery started out as a tool of assimilation, with ethnic immigrants wanting to look more "American."

The philosophy and techniques of cosmetic medicine didn't change much until the early twentieth century when, following World War I—the first war in which many soldiers survived their battlefield wounds—men returned home with disfiguring facial wounds that prevented them from working or going out in public. Much like the early Greeks and Romans, post-World War I cosmetic surgery patients were the disfigured who wanted to return to society or "pass" without being recognized. They desired form, function, and assimilation. One of the German surgeons of that era, Jacque Joseph, was known for his skills in reconstructing the complex facial wounds of veterans. He then translated his techniques and knowledge to alter characterizing facial features such as the noses of healthy, ethnic men and women who wanted to look "more German." Thus elective cosmetic surgery was born.

Joseph, a perceptive person and astute listener, knew that the goal of his new trade was to soothe the psyche of the patient, not to perfect the human form or achieve ultimate beauty. Americans were early proponents of cosmetic surgery, especially the Irish and Jewish immigrants of New York who wanted to alter their noses to look more "American." Other early adopters of cosmetic surgery were entertainers who wanted to hide their ethnic background, such as Fanny Brice, the Jewish comedienne immortalized by Barbara Streisand in *Funny Girl*, and criminals like John Dillinger who wanted to change their identity while on the run.

However, cosmetic surgery soon migrated from a tool of assimilation to a tool of separation. Since the beginning of recorded history, those who have felt they belong to the elite class of society used whatever they could to separate themselves from the underclass. From Nefertiti's facial makeup and Cleopatra's wine resin baths to the European upper crust's wigs and Asian empress's facial bleaching, the privileged class has always sought out physical signs to brand their status. Cosmetic medicine became an instrument of the privileged to flaunt their identity. In modern times, like many pop culture fads, the trend started with movie stars. Cosmetic medicine was used to separate the starlets from the common folk, and famous pin-ups like Marilyn Monroe were getting nose jobs. No longer was a vehicle for blending unnoticed into society, cosmetic surgery was used instead to help a person stand out.

Those undergoing surgery wanted to be more beautiful, developed, or youthful appearing than their competitors. This is where I believe plastic surgery took the wrong turn. In response to elitist demands, plastic surgeons began to offer physically altering treatments that were bold, large, and sure to emphasize sexual characterizing features of beauty and youth. Perhaps plastic surgeons of that era, many of whom combined competitiveness with a driven passion for their trade, like they still do today, were motivated to create greater changes that would be clearly and unmistakably identified. They set the standard for the profession.

Unfortunately, they got it wrong.

At conferences, the unspoken theme was to find the next best technique for pulling, tightening, or plumping in order to attain the ideals of beauty. This environment created conditions that celebrated heroic changes in the body and face. The field of cosmetic surgery went for the broad, obvious strokes and dismissed the subtleties that the human mind interprets as beauty.

The field of plastic surgery went for the broad, obvious strokes and dismissed the subtleties that the human mind interprets as beauty.

It became increasingly difficult to undergo a cosmetic procedure without others knowing it had been done. The psyche of one undergoing such a treatment recognized that yes, they looked better, but they also had to accept that others might recognize that "something had been done." They also had to accept a requisite healing period of at least six weeks to allow the ample bruising and swelling to subside before they could be seen again in public. Plastic surgery was even further limited to only those who could afford both the time and expense. It became a tool to reinforce class distinction, and the socially climbing elite tolerated the obvious level of cosmetic surgery alterations in order to better fit in with the upper crust.

It is however important to recognize that up to 1% of the population and 3-15% of those seeking out plastic surgery are afflicted with a distorted image of themselves, Body Dysmorphic Disorder (BDD). Much like anorexia nervosa, these people are never satisfied with their appearance. For the unfortunate victims of this disease plastic surgery may seem to be a cure for achieving the perfect body. Therefore they tend to be frequent visitors at multiple surgeons' offices. Yet, regardless of the intervention and/or how successful of an outcome from surgery, no treatment of body and form will suffice. It is important that this is recognized as a psychiatric medical condition and those who suffer from this are referred to the appropriate mental health counselors. As a plastic surgeon we are trained to identify BDD patients and to not operate on them. Unfortunately, sometimes we still see people who have had too many plastic surgery procedures. It appears that occasionally the BDD patient slips through and/or the surgeon dismisses the severity of the ailment.

Plastic surgery likely would have continued to speed blindly in the wrong direction had it not been for the discovery of the healing power of the world's most potent neurological toxin. Early research in the 1960s through 1980s identified that if used in micro doses, botulinum toxin safely and very effectively treated spastic muscle diseases around the eyes. Its therapeutic benefit expanded quickly to treating similar diseases of the neck and limbs in children with cerebral palsy. Soon it became known commercially as Botox and was used for multiple ailments including stuttering, facial tics, and swallowing disorders.

Botox, with its ease of use, quick onset, reversibility, and safety, became one of the most researched medicines in history. The drug's subtle wrinkle reducing facial altering effects forced cosmetic doctors who were stuck in the mindset that more is better to consider that maybe they'd gone wrong.

Unlike all previous cosmetic medical treatments, Botox offered aesthetically interested people a treatment that provided accurate and predictable results with little to no downtime and a very impressive safety record. Suddenly, the expectations, perceptions, and principles changed for all of cosmetic medicine. Patients now desired predictable and aesthetically pleasing outcomes with secrecy and little or no impact on their schedule. While not inexpensive, a Botox treatment was economically more accessible than surgical procedures which allowed the middle class to enter the market for the first time. As a result, the demand for Botox and similar cosmetic procedures skyrocketed.

Cracking a New Science of Beauty

For researchers, Botox was the model product for studying the effects of cosmetic changes on a person's psyche and behaviors. As scientists, we had been frustrated with our inability to study the true impact of our interventions. Traditional cosmetic procedures couldn't be tested with the standard scientific method, which compares two sets of people—one group that gets the experimental medicine and one that gets a placebo (neither they nor the researchers who give out the drug know which they received, which is why these are called double blind studies). We can't do that with plastic surgery because people would know if they did or didn't get plastic surgery and would therefore be biased to any questions researchers asked them afterwards.

The lack of rigorous testing is probably the primary reason plastic surgery did not progress like so many other fields of medicine. Plastic surgery techniques, training, and thinking had not significantly changed for a thousand years. The best treatments were based on the words of a few trusted master surgeons, but we had no scientific evidence to prove that what they said was true or really worked. Without study designs, we couldn't measure the effects that altering a face has on a person's attitude, self-esteem or other inner experience.

However, all of that changed with Botox.

Using precise unit measurements, we could now set up experimental studies to assess the effects of a cosmetic intervention with strict scientific standards. The intellectually curious trained in research now had a model in which to test theories.

Since patients have always told me that after their plastic surgery they believe others judge them more favorably and give them better treatment, I wanted to explore why. I was eager to better understand which parts

Primal perceptions: the subtleties that humans find attractive are often perceived on a subconscious level.

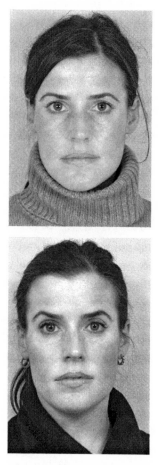

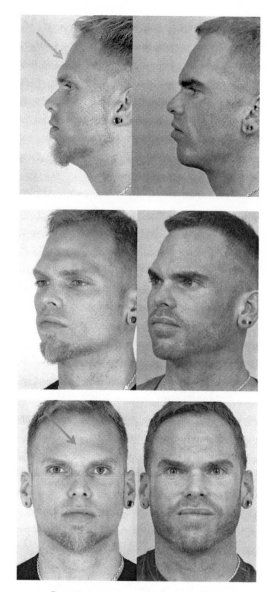

Botox treatment can be used to make the eyes appear more open friendly and inviting.

Prominent over-masculinizing brow reduced with nonsurgical treatment

of the face affect the impression that we project—what's the importance of raising the brows, widening the eyes, or lifting the corner of the mouth—and how can we heighten their positive effects?

In 2006, we published a study that revealed that those who underwent various minor facial plastic surgery procedures were judged more favorably by unknowing observers

(Dayan, Clark & Ho, 2004). We were fascinated with the results, but I wanted to know more. How did my surgical intervention affect the patient's improved perception, and what specific changes in the face caused the patient to project an improved impression?

I needed to study outside my field because the answers were not in plastic surgery. I began voraciously reading the neuropsychiatry literature and learned that the subtleties that humans find attractive are often perceived on a subconscious level. I was thrilled to discover a 2009 study conducted in Switzerland that revealed that barely detectable, minimal changes in features on an otherwise expressionless face can directly affect how that person is judged (Walker & Vetter, 2009). Based on images of people who had been digitally morphed, researchers found that, "Subtle and hardly perceivable differences in faces are powerful enough to cause judgments of personality."

This study was able to identify which parts of the face would translate into projecting a different image to others if slightly altered. The mouth was associated with social skill, the eyebrows and corners of the mouth to extroversion, the position of the mouth to aggression, and the nose to likeability. Wow! This means that altering a first impression for the better can be a relatively minor adjustment—major alterations are not necessary. And my days of studying evolutionary biology made it clear to me that these personality references were appealing to a human's primitive senses. Take the eyebrows, for example. A more arched less protruding eyebrow suggests someone is non-threatening and safe. It makes a person approachable.

Even the smallest change in our appearance can clue others into our personality. The Swiss scientists proved that a face can be made to look more likable, sociable, trustworthy, and extraverted. Their findings are further corroborated by other authors and scientists who have shown that mild changes in facial appearance will alter the impression one projects (Ekman, 1982; Laser &

> A mild change in facial appearance really does affect how one is perceived, and altering a first impression for the better can be a relatively minor adjustment.

Original face

Aggressiveness   Extroversion

Likeability   Risk seeking

Social skills   Trustworthiness

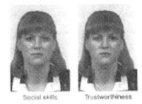

Mild barely detectable changes in a face can completely alter the personality one projects (Walker (2009) Journal of Vision.

> Our study recorded over 5,000 first impressions, making it one of the largest and most substantial first-impression studies to date. Our findings proved that mild, barely detectable changes in facial appearances can alter the first impression one makes.

Mathie, 1982). The profession was being turned upside down, and not everyone was ready for it.

These findings went against what was traditionally being taught and practiced in plastic surgery. Surgeons entrenched in developing more aggressive procedures to move major tissues and recreate faces in an idealized image said, "Hold it! Now the literature is telling us that all the patients needed to walk away happy are small changes?"

Botox, with its precise measurements and validated outcomes, continued to offer us an ideal model for further testing this curious and previously unexplored merging of appearance, psyche, and evolutionary behavior. Following in the footsteps of our study on the impact of facial plastic surgery on the appearance one projects, we were intrigued to more precisely evaluate the effects the mild changes in facial appearance can have on the impression one projects. We were able to narrow its effects to just one part of the face and use a control (untreated) group with which to compare. At last, we had a rigid and reproducible scientific model with which to test our ideas.

In 2008, we designed a new study in which we treated patients' eyebrow and forehead muscles with Botox, and then asked a group of unknowing observers to evaluate their standardized photos (Dayan et al., 2008). The observers were asked to make quick first-impression judgments of the people in each photograph based purely on appearance. The judging observers were not told anything about the patients or treatments and, like in our previous study, they never saw the same person's photo more than once. In total, we recorded over 5,000 first impressions, making this one of the largest and most substantial first-impression studies completed to date.

To be honest, when I looked at the photos side-by-side, I could hardly see a difference—and I have a trained eye for cosmetic changes. I was convinced that the untrained, unknowing observers would not be able to perceive a difference, and I was also curious about what my young, instinctive daughters would think, so I brought some of the pictures home. Of course I didn't tell them anything was done I just asked my kids which people in the photos were nicer, friendlier and happier. Without hesitation, the girls picked out the Botox treated patients!

This mirrored the findings of our observers.

After collating all the data, the patients who received Botox were found to be rated more attractive, more successful at dating, and more athletically successful. This was a fascinating finding that supports other research proving that mild, barely detectable changes in facial appearance can alter the first impression one makes.

I started to realize that plastic surgery training may be flawed. I had a eureka moment, recognizing for the first time that the slightest, most minimal changes in a face are the ones that alter the impression we give off! These effects weren't registering through our well-developed, highly sophisticated brain cortexes, but within the hidden and most primitive and animalistic parts of our brain. From an evolutionary perspective, mild facial alterations appealed to our most primal senses for detecting fear, sex, and competency, senses that developed over millions of years and that are critical to survival. Plastic surgery training told our over-analytical modern brains that the major lifting or tightening to achieve the idealized and often unnatural Adonis look that so commonly graced the cover of textbooks was right, but I was now saying that is wrong. That overdone look didn't appeal to the raw, primitive desires that make up the strong forces deep within every person's psyche. Our training didn't even acknowledge or mention the benefits of minor changes, because they weren't recognized. Or as one of my favorite professors used to always tell me, "The eye cannot see what the mind does not know."

I was more convinced than ever that the secret to projecting an attractive and positive first impression and subsequently enjoying all the fringe benefits bestowed onto the beautiful, involved subtle changes that not only increased a person's self-esteem, but spoke to the subconscious mind of the observer. It was about following the ideals of natural beauty that the master artists had always known. The future of cosmetic surgery would be a melding of science, medicine, psychology and art. But before going public with my new thinking, I needed further evidence and development. I couldn't launch a revolution based on one study; I had to show how it could have a bigger impact beyond plastic surgery.

Therefore, in addition to our findings from the Botox first-impression study, we evaluated the effects of other cosmetic procedures on the first impression. In our next study, we looked at the effects of filling in the nasolabial folds (the lines that run from the side of the nose to the side of the mouth) with Restylane (Dayan, Arkins & Gal, 2010). Following the filler treatment, the changes were once again subtle. Yet, three months afterward, using the same model of our two previous studies, we asked unknowing observers to rate their first impression of our patients who received the filler. Once again, our findings were highly significant—even more so than our findings with Botox. Our filler patients received a significantly higher first impression rating in several categories, including perceived social skills, academic performance, attractiveness, success in dating, career performance, finance, athletics, and relationships.

> In another study, our patients received a significantly higher first impression rating in several categories, including perceived social skills, academic performance, attractiveness, success in dating, career performance, finance, athletics, and relationships.

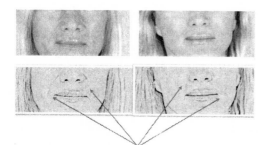

Hyaluronic filler before and after affords subtle changes that lead to a better first impression. The changes are difficult to see at first; however, when the photo is placed in contrast, the changes are more apparent. The conscious brain sees color; the subconscious brain sees the world through contrast.

Therefore, I now could positively report, based on credible scientific evidence, that Botox, filler treatments, and facial plastic surgery can all be strategically used to enhance important physical features, allowing one to project a more favorable first impression. However, the key point that had been missed by a generation of plastic surgeons is that the change imparted is subtle and barely perceivable.

It was finally clear to me that two fields of science—plastic surgery and neuropsychiatry—were becoming unified. The subconscious mind can and will detect and appreciate the mild natural changes of the face, resulting in a better impression, but there was one more component that still needed to be woven into the mix—self-esteem. I couldn't rest until I understood how our emotional psyche factored into appearance-related changes from plastic surgery. There was a large body of scientific evidence in behavioral and evolutionary psychology that linked self-esteem and appearance, but the ability to physically alter a face with plastic surgery and then quantify its effects on emotional well-being was yet to be explored.

The Life-Changing Effect of Feeling Good

A few years back, a patient of mine who had been coming in for Botox treatments every four months like clockwork came to the office a month early. Surprised, I mentioned that it had been only three months and asked her what was going on. It wasn't good news. She told me she had been diagnosed with breast cancer and was scheduled to undergo a series of tests and treatments. Then came the next surprise, before starting down that road, she wanted to get her Botox. I had suspected that Botox had been helping her with more than just reducing wrinkles. Sure enough, it made her feel better about herself, and she needed it now more than ever. Fortunately, all of her treatments went well and she survived her cancer.

In a related story, one of my well-to-do, high-fashion patients recently came in for a visit and told me she'd been sentenced to jail time for fraud. What a shocker! I would never have imagined that she was committing criminal acts. She told me she had come to terms with it and was headed off to a minimum-security prison for eighteen months. Yet, prior to going to jail, she wanted to get her filler treatments. Wow, I thought. She was headed to a women's prison in a remote part of Kentucky and would have no access to the outside world. There wasn't anyone inside she needed to impress with subtle changes to her physical attributes. Clearly, she was doing the cosmetic enhancements for no one but herself, because they made her feel better. It was something she could do to make her ordeal more bearable.

Still another example of how cosmetic medicine impacts self-esteem comes from early in my career, when I met with a rambunctious young lady from a small town in Wisconsin who had been born with a cleft lip/palate and deformed nose. Her lip had been repaired when she was a baby, but now she was in middle school and having some difficulty with her breathing from her nose. I treated her breathing problems and she improved, but neither she nor her mother mentioned or seemed bothered by her disfigured nose and lip. They didn't seem to prevent her from her winning, tomboy ways—she went on to be an All-State track star in high school and periodically her mother would send me clippings of her accomplishments from the local newspaper. She went to college on an athletic scholarship and thrived, doing well studying marketing. But when she came to the office just as she was about to graduate from college, I could tell she was down. She admitted that she didn't feel pretty because of her scarred and distorted lip and nose. I sensed her defeated attitude and inner deflation. She now identified more with her feminine side and was concerned that her appearance would hinder her success in a career and with men. She had become self-conscious about her looks and asked if there was anything I could do to help. I told her that I could improve the appearance of her nose and further camouflage the scars in her lip, but it would require surgery. I would need to take cartilage from her rib, carve it into a skeletal structure that would represent her nose, and then mold it in place under her nasal skin. I would have to cut out the scars of her lip and re-sew the

> Our research has clearly shown that subtle changes made within the guidelines of what human beings have evolved to find attractive are the key to making someone project a more favorable impression.

ends back together in a different geometric shape. Finally, I told her that when all was said and done her face would appear more natural and proportionally correct, but we could never achieve perfection. I needed to make sure she was well aware of the procedures and understood the outcomes. She thought about it for a few days and then called back and said, "Yes, I'm ready." I did the surgery and it went as planned.

Two years later she moved to New York City and started a job in advertising. Last Christmas, she came in to say hello with her mom. She walked in fashionably dressed, confident, and with purpose. Her external appearance had changed as well; she now wore long dark hair, a subtle hint of lipstick and makeup, a perfect manicure with dark maroon nail polish, and a large diamond engagement ring. She was all lady, and she and her mom couldn't wait to tell me about her new beau and upcoming wedding. They were in town

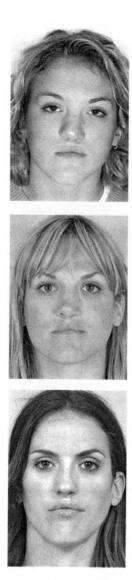

Two nose operations allowed a young tomboy with a cleft lip and palate nose deformity to appear and more importantly feel more feminine.

shopping for dresses. I was bowled over by the memory of that feisty little girl who grew into a high school track star and then a young woman with new priorities and desires. What a transformation. Late last year, they sent photos from her wedding with an arrow pointing to her nose and mentioning how much they appreciated my involvement. That photo sits in my office, another reminder that I have the best job in the world.

All of these patients sought out a plastic surgeon for so much more than an alteration in their appearance.

Our research has clearly shown that subtle changes made within the guidelines of what human beings have evolved to find attractive are the key to making someone project a more favorable impression. The next step was to tackle the chicken or the egg question.

We needed to discover *how* mild facial changes caused a person to create a better first impression—is it the physical alteration from the treatment itself, or is there a psychological transformation within the patient that results in him/her projecting a more favorable impression? I had always suspected that the perceived better treatment from others is not solely due to a physically improved appearance, but the result of the patient's reinvigorated self-esteem, which manifests as a more positive attitude.

I heard stories from my patients every day about how much better they felt about themselves after plastic surgery, but how much better, and why? What impact did that have on their lives? If I could get those answers, our profession could expand cosmetic treatments that could help many people from all walks of life with a variety of both medical and cosmetic concerns. From cancer survivors and trauma victims to under-developed children, aging housewives, and over-the-hill executives, all would benefit if we could tell them with accuracy how much and exactly what kind of benefit they can expect from a cosmetic treatment. The precise treatments and doses of what would be best for an individual could be determined with better-designed studies. Up to then, I'd been struggling to understand what impact my interventions were truly having on a person's self-esteem and well-being. Cosmetic plastic surgery was portrayed as a superfluous, non-serious, and non-academic field. I wanted to change that and better explain what we were achieving and why. All surgeons know wonderful stories of changing lives by erasing a defect on a face or body. And studies have backed this up. Women polled, after undergoing plastic surgery, felt a significant increase in self-power and were more productive at their jobs (Foustanos, Pantazi & Zavrides, 2007). All plastic surgeons recognize the power cosmetic treatments can have on someone's life, but because surgery is so variable from one person to the next and no two surgeries are performed in exactly the same way, it was difficult to organize those observations into meaningful information. We needed a different model, one with standardized treatments and protocols.

> It's very probable that those who undergo a variety of different cosmetic treatments— from chemical peels and nose jobs to liposuction—gain self-esteem, a sense of empowerment, are happier at work, and likely more satisfied in their home lives as well.

Once again, we turned to Botox to test our theories. Initial reports showed that patient satisfaction rates for those getting Botox were routinely above ninety percent, and this was impressive. A drug with that kind of a success rate was sure to catch on, but its popularity and growth had exceeded even the wildest expectations. Something else was going on to fuel its meteoric rise. We had already proven in an earlier study that those who get Botox treatments make a better first impression, so it made sense that patients were reporting that they received more favorable treatment from others after receiving Botox. I felt compelled to investigate this effect further.

Did people treat these patients better because they physically looked friendlier and happier, or was it my patients' heightened feelings about themselves that resulted in them projecting a more positive appearance and personality? I was intrigued when I read early reports showing that Botox treatments alleviated symptoms of depression, and while this study was small and uncontrolled, it stimulated a spark that Botox can affect mood (Lewis & Bowler, 2009). To better answer this question, we conducted a pilot trial in 2009 to test our hypothesis that those who get cosmetic medical treatments feel better about themselves. In our study, we found that the women we treated with Botox showed a significant increase in their mood and quality of life two weeks after the treatment. Another finding that I found particularly interesting was that there was a drop in their mood three months after the treatment. We realized that this corresponded to the Botox wearing off at that time, and this further emphasized that while Botox is working, mood is elevated.

While these findings were interesting and encouraging, the pilot study wasn't a well-designed, blinded, randomized, or controlled trial. Both the patients and I knew they were getting the Botox and this may have biased them to be happier. So in 2010 we used rigorous standards to launch a new, double-blind, randomized, placebo-controlled study into the effects of Botox on self-esteem and quality of life (Dayan, Arkins, Patel & Gal, 2010). Patients randomly received Botox or placebo saline, and neither the patients nor I knew which was being injected. We asked the patients to fill out a questionnaire that measures self-esteem and quality of life prior to being treated and weeks after the treatment. In addition, many of the patients had never had Botox treatments before (we called them Botox naïve), and having these patients as part of the study proved very significant because we were able to evaluate how Botox benefited first-time users.

Our findings were significant and confirmed what we found in the pilot trial. In just about all categories, Botox patients experienced greater self-esteem and quality of life after their treatments than did placebo patients. This was breakthrough data, and it supported my thoughts that those who get Botox not only project a better first impression, but also feel better about themselves and enjoy a better quality of life. Another highly interesting finding was that following the treatment those who never had Botox before had a much greater spike in their self-esteem (two times larger) than those who have had Botox in the past, and although, not below their baseline levels the Botox naïve patients' self- esteem dropped back down once the Botox wore off. Interestingly these patients' baseline levels of self-esteem to start with were lower than those who receive Botox routinely. This is a lot of information to process, but simply put, it means that those who get Botox routinely are happier, but those who never get Botox can really benefit in the short-term if they receive a treatment. This may be a way for someone to elevate his/her mood significantly if they really need it for an upcoming event.

> Cosmetic medical treatments may work to stimulate our brain's pleasure centers and elevate brain chemicals such as serotonin and dopamine that make us feel better about ourselves.

Although we proved that Botox improves one's quality of life, self-esteem, and projected first impression, these benefits are likely not exclusively limited to one product. Botox just gave us a scientific model in which to reliably test this theory. It's very probable that those who undergo a variety of different cosmetic treatments—from chemical peels and nose jobs to liposuction—all gain self-esteem, a sense of empowerment, are happier at work, and likely more satisfied in their home lives as well.

Cosmetic medical treatments may work to stimulate our brain's pleasure centers and elevate brain chemicals such as serotonin and dopamine that make us feel better about ourselves. However, this process isn't happening directly, with the chemicals or drugs passing into the brain, but rather *indirectly* when we look into the mirror and like what we see. Our satisfaction with the subtle changes triggers the pleasure response in the brain. There is also evidence that emotions are secondary to facial expression. In other words, if you squeeze your eyebrows together in a scowl, you actually start to feel angry, or conversely, if you smile, you induce happiness.

There's also evidence that persistently angry or sad emotions and facial expressions can lead to long-term changes in the face, which result in permanent wrinkles that become associated with these negative behaviors (Malatesta, Fiore & Messina, 1987). This means that a person who is consistently angry and always making an "angry face" may develop permanent scowl lines in his/her brow and forehead. Such features on a person face then just perhaps give off impressions that have real accuracy (Zebrowitz & Collins, 1997). In other words people who always look angry maybe really are angry!

> A cosmetic alteration that could stop anger, promote happiness, and prevent permanent wrinkles could have a significant and dramatic physiological, psychological, and behavioral impact.

Based on this physical-emotional connection, if we could lessen someone's ability to make an angry face by using a filler or Botox, theoretically we could reduce anger and the physiological ramifications to the body that come with an angry mood. If we can turn up the corner of the mouth slightly and promote a smile, perhaps this would launch a biofeedback response that affects the brain and makes one feel happier.

What a fantastic thought! A cosmetic alteration that could stop anger, promote happiness, and prevent permanent wrinkles could have a significant and dramatic physiological, psychological, and behavioral impact beyond making someone a bit more beautiful. I realized that when we take an active step in improving our appearance, we launch a powerful domino effect:

We see a more youthful reflection in the mirror, which makes us feel better;

This affects our brain chemistry, flooding us with feel-good serotonin and dopamine;

Feeling better, we stand taller, smile more, and unleash a cascade of physiological events and hormones throughout our bodies that trigger subtle, barely detectable changes in our appearance that make us not only feel better, but also look better.

This was my biggest "aha!" moment yet. I could confidently weave in the third strand and prove that the three fields of plastic surgery, neuropsychiatry, and behavioral psychology had to be unified to bring our patients the happiness and better quality of life they desire. Yes, plastic surgery will result in a physical change, but now we could prove that the physical change results in a measureable increase in self-esteem and a better first impression, which positively affects the judgment received from others.

The next step was figuring out how to put into practice this three-fold concept.

The Subliminal Difference

The Subliminal Difference philosophy consists of providing facial cosmetic treatments that naturally highlight the evolutionarily determined attractive features of the face and deemphasize those that detract, all below the detection of the conscious mind.

These subliminal changes affect the primitive and more influential subconscious mind. The key—and quantum shift from the traditional philosophy of plastic surgery—is that nobody other than the patient can detect that a treatment was done. If even the slightest hint of a procedure is obvious, whether it be a scar or lips that are too big, others would subconsciously read this as a tipoff that this person is a fake and actually hiding a genetic weakness. The person would be worse off than if they had done nothing at all.

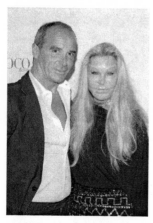

The Famed "Cat woman"

The above photographs show the subliminal difference approach in action. The patient was treated non-surgically over an eighteen-month period in which her weight remained constant. As the changes were subtle and gradual, we did not recognize the impression altering changes in her appearance, until she came in one day mentioning how much happier and better her life had become. She was commenting on how pleased she was with her treatments and believed she was looking better since becoming a patient. This prompted us to look back at her photographs to see if we could identify the differences. After closely studying her pictures and treatment regiment, it was then that I started to realize the power of gradual, small and subconsciously effective changes of the face. The upper one-third of her face was treated with Botox to create a slightly and barely noticeable raising of her brow, which reduced forehead wrinkles and opened the eyelid aperture—resulting in a subliminal message of friendliness and youthful fertility. Her eyelashes were enhanced with Latisse, further drawing attention to the eyes. Radiesse filler in the cheeks further accentuated the eyes and drew attention away from the lower third of the face. The lower third of the face was deemphasized and the width of the jaw was narrowed with Botox into the jaw muscles, allowing the lips, which are subtly augmented with Juvederm, to be further noticeable, but not distracting. The skin was homogenized, plumped and toned following a laser CO_2 treatment.

The result is a face that conveys femininity, youthfulness, and beauty while remaining subtle, natural, and within the context of her age.

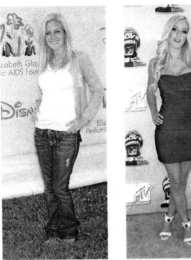
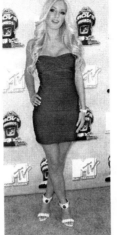

Heidi Montag, does she look better after all the plastic surgery? Many would say no.

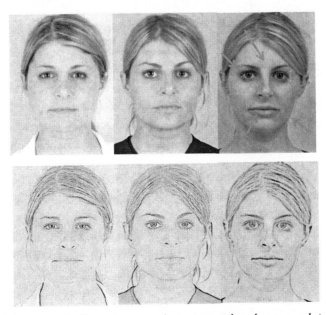

Subliminal changes in the face using an evolutionary guide to beauty result in a more attractive face. Fillers and neuromodulators were used to shape and beautify the face with two treatments. Contrast enhancement makes the changes more apparent to the conscious mind.

Those undergoing a subliminal difference treatment report to us that they have more self-confidence, an improved quality of life, and are treated more favorably by others.

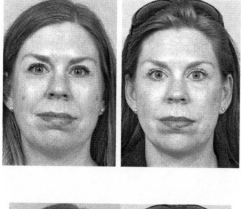

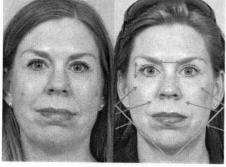

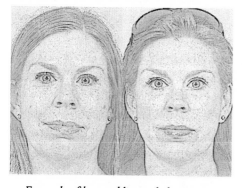

*Example of how subliminal changes can
and will alter the impression a face projects*

The subliminal difference isn't defined or limited to one type of procedure or product; rather, it is a philosophy to alter one's appearance within the context of an evolutionary guide to make a face naturally appear more attractive. Whether we use makeup, skin care, or medical treatments, enhancing nature's key areas of beauty can and will improve the first impression we project, boost self-esteem, and increase emotional well-being. We've proven it (Dayan & Arkins, 2012).

In plastic surgery, we are trained to be goal-oriented toward the traditional physical "ideals of beauty." In an attempt to see or recognize an improvement, there may have been a tendency for surgeons to push beyond what is natural. But I'm convinced that if we want to make someone appear better, we need to do fewer large changes and focus on the minor alterations that are barely detectable to the unknowing observer, yet fall within the evolutionary adaptive traits that stimulate the subconscious mind to interpret a face as beautiful.

Beyond "Cosmetic" Surgery

Although Botox, facelifts, and tummy-tucks have been branded a luxury for the vain, rich, and famous, by unifying the three fields of study we can now prove that subliminally designed treatments and cosmetic plastic surgery can play a much bigger role for many people from all backgrounds. When done in a natural and barely detectable manner, cosmetic treatments can give to so many the self-esteem and quality of life that has eluded or been taken from them. Yes, we can reduce wrinkles for those wanting to look younger, but we can also provide facial symmetry to stroke victims, reduce acne scars to disenfranchised youths, and replace noses destroyed by skin cancer. Once the fantasies of sci-fi movies, surgical facial transplants are now giving hope to the severely disfigured. Breast implants, while considered by some a fake-looking choice for would-be beauty queens, are also a femininity-saving procedure for the thousands of women who undergo a mastectomy for breast cancer.

> Whether we use makeup, skin care, or medical treatments, enhancing nature's key areas of beauty can and will improve the first impression we project, boost our self-esteem, and increase our emotional well-being.

A fifty-year-old, postmenopausal breast cancer survivor can live without her breast, but it's certainly a critical quality of life and cosmetic issue. The difficulty comes when we start to explore and better understand the quality of life issue inherent to cosmetic procedures.

Where do we draw the line between what is and what isn't cosmetic? Is treating female baldness cosmetic? How about HIV victims who experience facial wasting? What about obese adolescents? All of these individuals can undergo treatments to alleviate the cosmetic effects of these conditions, none of which are necessary for survival, but all of which have cosmetic and quality of life implications. As we begin to study and further measure the benefits of cosmetic medicine to the individual's psyche, the lines between functional and cosmetic become even more blurred.

In my practice, I now focus more on the evolutionary adaptive traits of beauty and their relationship to cosmetic medical treatments, the human psyche, and the subsequent behaviors in our patients and those that encounter them. I've expanded my view of plastic surgery beyond the two-dimensional lenses of form and function. I now see it in three dimensions, adding in the workings of the primal, subconscious mind.

More and more people consider cosmetic treatment as normal and acceptable as coloring their hair. Cosmetic surgery is no longer a boutique subspecialty of medicine for elitists who want to separate themselves from the pack—today, cosmetic medicine is a field of study breaking new ground in improving quality of life issues for many Americans. Cosmetic medicine gives victims of physical or emotional trauma a path for returning to society. And on a broader scale, it gives people of all backgrounds additional tools for improving their quality of life and satisfying one of the most primal human instincts—wanting to look our best.

We're just starting to see the exciting effects that cosmetic medicine can have on our society. Beyond projecting a more favorable first impression, millions of Americans can enjoy a better quality of life, which triggers the positive ripple effect of bringing a more positive approach to life at home, at work, and into the world.

I predict that in the coming years a new field of study will emerge, for now let's call it "Aestimoaesthetic biology," a science that focuses on the relationship between facial/body aesthetics and mood, health and well-being. I believe it will appeal to and attract experts from the established fields of dermatology, plastic surgery, facial plastic surgery occuloplastic surgery, behavioral psychology, evolutionary biology, neuropsychiatry and even those traditionally regarded outside of science to include fashion and style make-up and skin care experts. I predict this will spawn a new field of medicine, "Aestimoaesthetic medicine." A specialty that will include thinking, training, products and procedures, that prevent, mitigate and cure diseases through the influence of both the mind and body with aesthetics. I believe this new field of medicine will expand the indications of aesthetic treatments to help people with a variety of ailments from all walks of life. Negative veils of vanity pinned on the natural urges to appear more beautiful will be shed. As the Renaissance was to European culture, medieval shackles still evident today on the desire to be and act on being beautiful will be shattered. Greek and Romans viewed beauty as an abstract perfect form although never completely achievable its pursuit encouraged, 'Aestimoaesthetic" medicine will bring enlightenment back to a post-modern generation. When will all this occur, I am not entirely sure but the inertia is unstoppable.

CHAPTER 12

CASHING IN

"He [Aristotle] used to say that personal beauty was a better introduction than any letter."

—Diogenes Laertius, *The Lives and Opinions of the Eminent Philosophers* (ca. 200 A.D.)

By now, you're probably convinced that our primitive wiring controls a lot, if not most of our behavior involving attraction. But if you've still got any doubts, just turn on the TV and watch an episode of "The Bachelor." That should clinch it. My kids love this reality show.

The other night I sat and watched an episode with them—well, at least as much as I could over the racket as they cheered on their favorite femme fatale. The premise is that one very eligible, wealthy, and attractive bachelor dates a dozen beautiful women and in each episode narrows down the group by selecting those whom he wants to continue dating; the others are eliminated. It's very

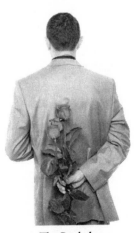

The Bachelor

dramatic as he awards those he selects with a rose through a very drawn-out process while all the women stand at attention in their evening gowns. If that isn't enough, the women, who are all in competition with each other, live together. This bees' nest of females with exploding hormones and emotions is then probed and prodded with questions from the very inquisitive host, allowing their most primitive urges and reactions to be exposed to millions of viewers. They scheme, outmaneuver, block, and sell out each other as they each compete to win the beau. The fact that this show is a hit is the best evidence yet that we have evolved so little over the last 100,000 years!

Solid evidence shows us that those who are considered more attractive and beautiful win more advantages in life. As early as primary school, the best-looking kids receive better grades and are treated better, and this continues through adolescence and beyond. For women, the economics of being beautiful are directly correlated to whom they choose as a mate. Like it or not, beauty is like a commodity that women can trade in for a more resourceful, wealthy man, and women will compete with each other for the man with the most assets. It explains why Jackie Kennedy moved on to the even wealthier Aristotle Onassis and Princess Di traded up for Dodi Fayed. I know this sounds callous and sexist, but natural selection and evolution are only concerned with survival of the species. Mother Nature is insensitive to the social, political, or religious ethos of the day—if a woman is biologically driven to give birth to genetically fit children and be able to protect them until they become self-sufficient, she will be motivated to find the perfect mate, even if that means pushing a friend out of the way. This may be why women are particularly concerned about what they wear and how it measures up to what her friends are wearing on an important night out, and why a woman may be quick to put down a potential competitor.

> Beauty is like a commodity that women can trade in for a more resourceful, wealthy man, and women will compete with each other for the man with the most assets.

Why Women Feel Uneasy Around Beautiful Women

As we learned in Chapter Six, women know that the most beautiful woman in the room has the mate-capturing advantage. She also intuitively knows that her man will probably find her less desirable after viewing a more attractive woman. This phenomenon, coined the "Farrah effect," explains why some women are threatened when their partner spends a night out with the boys at the local gentleman's club. However, the effect is time limited, and a man soon returns to his baseline ratings of female attractiveness.

Yet, as TV's "Real Housewives" reality shows prove, finding a rich, handsome man doesn't necessarily correlate with happiness. Most evidence points to happiness as innate, self-generated, and highly dependent on how one feels about his/her appearance

Men are acutely aware that a woman will preferentially choose to date and subsequently have sex with a man who wears a Rolex wristwatch rather than a Burger King outfit.

(Baumeister et al., 2003). And as a woman's physical assets wane, she may feel pressure to find another way of keeping her resource-providing man interested, especially if he is wealthy or attractive. Some highly successful and symmetric men may feel an urge to wander once the kids are past the age of seven and relatively self-sufficient. Although our natural human instincts are appropriate for a lifespan of forty years in the harsh, primitive environment in which our species developed, such behavior today clashes with the rules of a stable society, not to mention our cultural and religious values. In Western society, we have religious doctrines and divorce laws in place to discourage and penalize such behavior.

Men strive to acquire assets and show them off because those with social, political, and financial resources have access to more attractive and likely more genetically fit women—Hugh Hefner has three girlfriends and Donald Trump's third wife is twenty-four years younger than he is. Men are acutely aware that a woman will preferentially choose to date and subsequently have sex with a man who wears a Rolex wristwatch rather than a Burger King outfit (Townsend & Levy, 1990). Once a man achieves wealth, he realizes he has increased his chances of getting a more attractive mate (Montoya, 2008). However, a man who isn't able to provide resources is at a much greater risk of losing his partner to another more able provider. And if his mate accumulates her own resources, she may no longer feel dependent on him, which heightens his risk of losing her as well. This may be why men feel threatened by women who make more money than they do, and why women in high-powered positions often marry men who have even higher statuses.

More than half of corporate hiring managers surveyed said that they advised job-seekers to spend at least as much money on improving their appearance as they did on perfecting their resume.

The Attractive Edge

For both sexes, being more attractive means a better chance for being hired for a job (Collins & Zebrowitz, 1995). *Newsweek*, in a special report entitled "The Beauty Advantage," surveyed corporate hiring managers and found that more than fifty percent of them advised job-seekers to spend at least as much money on improving their appearance as they did on perfecting their resume. Yet, the first impression projected at that interview must be consistent with the job. An attractive twenty-something in a tight-fitting summer dress is more likely to get an offer to be on a new "Baywatch" series than be coveted for a boardroom position.

Until a man's mind evolves past the Pleistocene era, an attractive woman focused on climbing the corporate ladder may want to consider dressing in a manner that deemphasizes her sexual traits.

Standards of what is ideal physically, socially, and professionally may also vary based on geography. In a non-scientific poll we conducted in 2006, we asked fifty women in Los Angeles and fifty women in Chicago at what age they thought a woman looks her best. In Los Angeles, the surveyed women said age twenty-six, but in Chicago, our respondents said thirty-five. These results were very interesting, because most studies evaluating the male mind find that a man defines the ideal age for feminine beauty to be about 24 (Buss et al., 2000; Johnston et al., 2003). This is close to the answer given by our responders in Los Angeles, and we figured that the reason for placing a female's peak at a younger age in L.A. is that success in the ever-prevalent entertainment industry is very dependent on appearance. And in that warmer environment, the clothing styles and year-round bathing suits that accentuate the feminine figure allow a younger and more fertile woman to more likely be noticed. However, in Chicago, the weather and professional environment would be more selective to a slightly more mature woman. So, a thirty-something woman who wants to live in a location in which she would be considered in her prime is more likely to find it in the Midwest. However, she'll have to invest in a parka for the winter months.

Although being attractive is important to being hired in the corporate world, for both a man and woman a female's attractiveness may be an obstacle to achieving higher managerial positions (Lyness & Heilman, 2006; Lyness & Thompson, 1997). Women are held to a higher standard before being promoted to a position that requires management and delegation. Therefore, until a man's mind evolves past the Pleistocene era, an attractive woman focused on climbing the corporate ladder may want to consider dressing in a manner that deemphasizes her sexual traits. It might be advantageous for her to avoid wearing her hair down or a tight, formfitting dress with a plunging neckline to her next review.

But regardless of the employment level, being attractive is worth more money in the workplace. One study even put percentages on the beauty premium. In an article published in *The American Economic Review*, professors affiliated with the University of Texas and Michigan State University revealed some interesting findings on the labor force (Hamermesh & Biddle, 1994). They reviewed men and women from the United States and Canada and found that being more attractive

Going from below average to above average in appearance results in an income gain that most studies equate to an extra one-and-a-half years of schooling!

than average resulted in earning more money and appearing plain resulted in earning less than average-looking people.

Going from average to below average in appearance shifted earnings downward, and the plainness penalty is five to ten percent larger than the beauty premium. In other words, when it comes to earning power, there is more of a detriment to being unattractive than there is a benefit to being good-looking, but the benefit is still there. Going from below average to above average in appearance results in an income gain that most studies equate to an extra one-and-a-half years of schooling! The researchers concluded that the only way to account for the income differences across all the occupations in their study was "pure . . . discrimination based on beauty and stemming from employer/employee tastes."

This beauty benefit can be seen for men in the legal profession as well. In a 1998 study published in the *Journal of Economics*, the graduation photos of over 4,400 attorneys were followed for more than fifteen years, and it turned out that those who were judged more attractive based on their photo were earning more money (Biddle & Hamermesh, 1998). The attractive male lawyers were also more likely to bill at a higher rate and work in the private sector where their good looks were worth more financially. Attractive men were also more likely to obtain partnership early. Perhaps these better-looking attorneys were more likely to be successful in front of judges, or maybe their attractive looks resulted in a marketing advantage when attaining new clients.

> We seem to instinctively prefer stronger and more dominant-appearing leaders.

Handsome CEOs

Researchers have also discovered that taller-looking men are likely to make more money and achieve greater heights in the corporate world (Collins & Zebrowitz, 1995), and as we saw in Chapter Four, other studies show that most CEOs are tall with a full head of hair.

But can a company's success be predicted by the appearance of the CEO alone?

This was the question posed by a study that asked college students to rate the photographs of CEOs from the top 25 and bottom 25 on the *Fortune* 1000 list of companies. They ranked the men in the photos on categories of power (facial maturity, competence, and dominance), warmth (likability and trustworthiness), and overall leadership qualities (Rule & Ambady, 2008). The company's revenues and profits were then examined against the students' ratings, and what do you think they found? Lo and behold, the 25 most profitable companies are led by CEOs that rated highly in power and leadership qualities based on their facial appearance. These men were *not* rated highly in warmth categories, which show that although likability and trustworthiness are important to leadership, we seem to instinctively prefer stronger and more dominant-appearing leaders. These first impressions are mediated deep within a very primitive part of the brain (Rule et al., 2011).

Plastic Surgery and Job Success

If the best-looking people seem to rise to the top, is there an economic and professional advantage to getting a nose job, breast augmentation, or chin implant? A study published in *Aesthetic Plastic Surgery* found that those who underwent plastic surgery felt it was a good investment in their career and made them feel more productive at work (Foustanos, et al., 2007). Others have also noted that those who get plastic surgery believe they achieve greater acceptance at work (Newell, 2000).

In our own studies on cosmetic surgery and self-esteem, our trials showed that those who get Botox are more satisfied with their ability to be productive and successful at work (Dayan, et al., 2008; Dayan, et al., 2010). Clearly, feeling better about the way we look correlates with higher self-esteem, which results in an ability to better tolerate negative situations, be more confident, and take more risks. Additionally, women who believe they are attractive are likely to earn more money, and men who feel attractive are likely to be promoted further. Elevated self-esteem is associated with excelling in the workplace and having a happier disposition both in and out of work (Boehm & Lyubomirsky, 2008).

Being better-looking and taller, having more hair, or possessing ideal measurements will get you in the door, but if you fail to be as good as you advertise, you'll be penalized more severely than those without such attractive qualities. You'll be held to a higher standard. Therefore, in the short-term, cosmetic treatments and the high self-esteem that goes along with them may open a door to new opportunities, but it may be short lived. The key to being professionally successful is based on so much more than physical appearances alone. You have to deliver the expected results or risk being put at a disadvantage sooner.

In an experiment set up to mimic everyday exchanges between people, participants took part in a game about cooperation (Mulford, Orbell, Shatto & Stockard, 1998). Researchers discovered that people were more willing to cooperate and engage with those who were more attractive. Being perceived as attractive brings opportunities for productive encounters and others want to interact with those they see as attractive, even it if comes at some expected cost. What was most intriguing to me about this report was that one's self-assessment of his or her attractiveness played a very important role in determining "who gets what." In fact, for women, it was very important for them to think of themselves as attractive in order to make more money. For each point higher on an eleven-point scale of attractiveness that others rated a woman attractive, she was likely to earn an additional fifty cents, but for each point higher a woman rated *her* own attractiveness on the 11-point scale, she was likely to profit eighty-six cents.

> Women who believe they are attractive are likely to earn more money.

What a finding! If a woman thinks she is attractive, she can do seventy percent better!

This behavior didn't exist for men, but it clearly showed that a woman's positive, attractive self-image gives her real financial gains that can be measured in the laboratory.

Regardless of culture, those who are beautiful are initially likely to gain an advantage when it comes to getting a job, making money, or being judged in court. If they can also deliver everything it takes to do the job well, being smart and projecting an attractive image will likely get them much further in their career. An attractive individual oozes confidence, stands tall, speaks well, and is more likely to gain prolonged favor and success. And while not everyone is born with raw beauty, attractiveness is very much under our control.

The (In) Justice of Beauty

Attractiveness also seems to give you an edge in court.

Being more attractive brings greater success in legal proceedings and gets you more favorable treatment from a jury or judge (Sarwer, Grossbart & Didie, 2003). However, being attractive in court can also be a detriment, especially if it involves a case in which an

> Being attractive gets you more favorable treatment from a jury.

attractive person took advantage of a less attractive person. This has been found in cases of money swindling or in a man taking advantage of a woman. Our instincts tell us that attractive men are not supposed to prey on women, and this primal attitude carries all the way into the court system (Aloha, 2010). And this goes for women as well—why do you think Casey Anthony wore plain clothing and hairstyles and little, if any, makeup during her trial for the murder of her two-year-old daughter? Her attorneys knew that the more motherly and homely she appeared, the better chance she had of being found innocent (the jury found her not guilty of murder).

The same goes for dashing swindlers. It's almost as if they were given an advantage in life by being good-looking, and juries punished them for using it to take advantage of a less fortunate person.

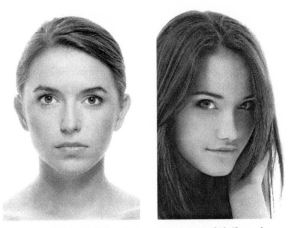

A woman with her hair up is perceived differently than than a woman with her hair down.

Beauty Sells

Do you think you are more likely to buy coffee from a highly attractive woman like Angelina Jolie, or someone not as strikingly beautiful, like Joan Cusack? What if they were selling a hair care product or perfume? The reason men may be more inclined to buy another beer from the vixen behind the bar in a skimpy pair of shorts may have more to do with her physical assets than her pouring skills.

> Attractive people are hired and promoted because they make us feel good.

Likewise, the strutting, confident man in a gritty outfit at the hardware store might be more likely to upsell a set of tools to a thirty-something mom than would a thin, nerdy high school kid with pimples.

One reason attractive people are hired and promoted is that they make us feel good. In a split second, viewing an attractive face can trigger positive emotions and stimulate pleasure centers in our brain. We're wired to want to associate with attractive people both personally and professionally. Attractive people prime us to feel positive, and we then assume they will prime others positively, too.

In a 2005 study, attractive faces flashed on a screen for one second increased the mental processing and reaction time for positive words more than unattractive faces did (Olson & Marshuetz, 2005). Pretty people prime our brains to find something positive or good, and this likely translates into selling better. For a hiring manager, it's common sense to want an attractive frontline person to have the first interaction with the customer. It looks good for the product and for the business. The reasons are obvious and biological.

However, being attractive needs to be consistent with what is being sold. Yes, attractive women are more noticeable to both males and females, but their value as endorsers is highly relevant on what they are selling. If the product advertised can be naturally associated with the endorser, an attractive model may make the consumer more receptive to the message. However, if the product has no association with the attractiveness of the model, there may be no effect, or possibly, a negative outcome (Baker & Churchill, 1977).

In a study testing this theory, men were shown an advertisement for coffee featuring both attractive and unattractive models, and the unattractive models produced much higher behavioral intentions than the attractive ones. In other words, men were more likely to want to buy the coffee from the less attractive woman because her appearance made more sense in relation to that product. However, the reaction was reversed when the product was perfume. The attractive model proved to be more persuasive than her unattractive counterpart in convincing the men to buy the perfume.

The SAFE Way of Getting Ahead

The four senses common to all humans—sex, appetite, fear, and ego (SAFE)—have been deeply woven into our inner core over millions of years of evolution. While they can be suppressed and repressed, they can't be denied. They are visceral, from the gut, and necessary to our survival. When any one of these senses is tugged, we can't help but take notice. Our intellect may decide to pass on the opportunity, but our primitive mind will want to at least process and evaluate the information. Based on everything I've learned and witnessed, I believe that if you want to capture someone's attention or persuade them to do something, you'll succeed by appealing to one of these four senses. Whether you are selling a product, engaging someone in conversation, looking for a quick response to your email, or desiring a person's attention, you are more likely to capture what you want by appealing to his or her SAFE factors. Human beings simply can't help being engaged when one of these four senses is stimulated.

> We can't help being engaged when one of our SAFE senses—sex, appetite, fear, and ego— is stimulated.

Biologically speaking, our sole purpose on Earth is to procreate and foster a genetic code that is better adapted to survive. Of all the visceral urges, sex is perhaps our strongest and most difficult to ignore. There is a reason why heads turn when an attractive person walks past and why pornography is a ten- to fourteen-billion-dollar-a-year business (*Forbes*). If you want to incorporate one of the SAFE drives into your appeal or strategy, you must know how to deliver it within the right context, or it will lose its value, or worse, work against you. One of the best examples of this is sex in advertising.

Sex grabs attention and stirs emotions, but does it sell?

Studies tell us yes and no—it depends on the product. Advertisements with sexual content get higher visual recall and recognition scores (Reid & Soley, 1983), but that doesn't mean the person viewing the ad is any more likely to buy the product. In a highly sexual ad, the viewer's attention and processing of information is devoted to the sexual content and messaging, leaving little brainpower left for perceiving the advertised information. In other words, we focus on the sexual content of the advertisement so much that it detracts from seeing the message of the product and/or brand. While an ad alluding to sex is likely to be remembered, the actual product is less likely to be remembered than one advertised in a non-sexual ad.

> In a highly sexual ad, the viewer's attention is so devoted to the sexual content that there's no brainpower left for perceiving information about the product.

Sexual promotions work best when there's a close link between sexual content and the product being sold. If a sexually charged ad is produced for selling condoms or intimate oils, it will be more effective than an ad filled with sexual innuendo that's trying to sell hamburgers.

Appetite, the second SAFE sense, aligns with hunger, a powerful primitive urge that will motivate people to do just about anything if it's taken to the extreme. Television producers and advertisers are well aware of the strength of this drive, and it shows in all the chef competitions, food shows, and food advertisements aired just before the dinner hour. Even more unscrupulous are the food ads that prey on children—forty-nine percent of the advertising on Saturday morning TV is devoted to food products (Batada, 2008).

Our local coffee, ice cream shops, and grocery stores also cater to our hunger drive by tempting us with samples of biscotti, the latest gooey chocolate treats, and easy-to-prepare snacks and entrees we're tempted to stock up on at home. Once our hunger is awakened, we want to keep tasting and are more likely to listen to what the vendor has to say. After we're satiated, however, our attention turns off and the clerk may have a more difficult time persuading us. So, a successful sales pitch with food means engaging with a receptive, eager, and compliant audience early in their sampling trip. Even non-food products can benefit from appealing to the hunger drive. Offering food is one of the best ways to capture another's attention, and the sweeter the better. The human urge for the quick and powerful energy boost of sugar is hard-wired and tough to resist. Satisfying people's appetite for irresistible foods is one of the quickest ways to open them up and allow deeper engagement, which is why food and drink are so often part of a first meeting.

Fear, another prewired sense critical to our survival, is processed swiftly in the brain because it's in our best interest to quickly size up a threatening situation and act to avoid danger. The primitive human brain senses whether someone is trustworthy or not within microseconds—faster than any other character trait. If you can provoke someone's fear, they will be motivated to act. We see this in ads every day, from public service announcements about the dangers of cigarette smoking to commercials for house alarms. Fear is also a staple in politics, religion, and, in many cases, parenting.

Appealing to one's ego is also a very straightforward process. It's human nature to want to be validated and recognized, and most of us will rate the quality of something we've helped create more highly than something made by a random person. Whether it's an art project, our homes, or photos of our grandchildren, we tend to overvalue it compared to what others think of it. We also tend to rate ourselves more attractive than others do, and rate our importance to the success of a project greater than that of others. And if a project fails, we recuse ourselves of the blame more quickly than we excuse others. It's not in our nature to see ourselves as failures.

> The first step in validating and appealing to another's ego starts with listening—really listening.

The first step in validating and appealing to another's ego starts with listening—really listening. This is without a doubt one of the most difficult tasks to do. I challenge you today, in your next conversation with your spouse, another family member, co-worker, or the person on the plane sitting next to you, to try to ask questions and just listen without being quick to formulate what you are going to say. Really try to understand the other person. What are his or her desires, fears, and passions? Try to engage them warmly and affectionately. This is crucial when meeting someone for the first time. If you want people to find you attractive, they need to feel attractive, and by smiling at them you will not only increase how they feel about themselves, but also alter how they perceive and treat you (Jones, DeBruine, Little, Conway & Feinberg, 2006; Jones et al., 2005). Afterward, with a better understanding of who this person is and having captured their attention, frame your conversation in such a way that you can adjust your argument, sales pitch, or conversation to their ego desires.

If you are in sales, it's not about what you want to say, but what your customer wants to hear. Corporate executives and sales representatives seem to have the hardest time with this concept. From CEOs on down, I'm amazed at how often a company will not think through a process or product from their customer's point of view. I recently sat in on a health business seminar in Paris and listened to thirty CEOs boast about the greatness of their companies. None of them mentioned how their product was important to me, the doctor, or to the patient. If they were focusing on appealing to the financial people in audience, they did a good job, but they weren't trying to engage those who consume and benefit from their products. Taking the time to listen and gather true insight about another person's passions will allow you to gain better appeal. Regardless of the situation or culture, being considerate of another person's interests and desires will not only bring you new friends, but also help you prosper.

And if a relationship falls short of expectations or fails, the first question to ask yourself is, "what could I have done differently?" The easy and most common reaction following a dispute is to immediately blame the other person, but that only sets you up for future disappointments. The failure of any relationship rests within an inability to effectively communicate. This includes most importantly listening and understanding the other's desires and secondly expressing what you want and need within a compromising framework. By honestly admitting to what you want and need and then asking if it is acceptable the other person will be less guarded and more willing to cooperate. When true emotions, feelings or desires are hidden, cryptically messaged or veiled within intimidating behaviors the relationship, whether professionally or personally, is doomed for insignificance.

These four essential senses work subconsciously, overriding our conscious, more mannered behaviors. By appealing to them we can bypass another's defenses and reach their soft, authentic inner core. The SAFE senses are perhaps the strongest and most reliable threads that connect us all. As much as our cultural, political, religious, and personality differences get touted, the one prevailing theme I've learned from my explorations is that we all have more in common than we think, and it is these commonalities that can be used to unite us. Regardless of whether the context is nation building, neighborly relations, or selling lemonade on the street, think SAFE and you will always find a route that can bring success.

"Cashing In" doesn't just refer to beauty and money, but involves recognizing and mastering all the visceral senses so that you can communicate your feelings, wishes, and desires more richly and effectively.

CHAPTER 13

WHAT'S IT ALL MEAN?
CONCLUSION

"Let no one ever come to you without leaving better and happier."
—Mother Teresa

As the genetic beneficiary of two divergent cultures, Barack Obama seems to have inherited the best of both worlds. Tall, athletic, intelligent, and eloquent, he burst onto the scene as an Illinois State Senator in 1997 and rapidly infatuated and warmed the hearts of millions on his rise toward becoming arguably the most powerful man in the world. Italian icon Sophia Loren, rated one of the top twenty-five actresses of all time by the American Film Institute, is a knockout natural beauty with large eyes, highly symmetric facial features, an hourglass figure, and gorgeous smile. At seventy-eight, she still exudes class and sophistication and gains elegance with each passing year. Award-winning actor and overall hunk Brad Pitt is one generation's biggest heartthrob. His exceedingly handsome features and physique not only put him on the cover of *People* as the "Sexiest Man Alive" twice, but also define male attractiveness.

While all three of these notables share the common ground of physical beauty, it is their undeniable attractiveness that has given them a decided advantage in their quest for success.

The appeal of attractiveness also links them to others who by objective standards may not seem so easy on the eyes: Winston Churchill, Abraham Lincoln, Steve Jobs, Albert Einstein, Margaret Thatcher, Golda Meir, and Eleanor Roosevelt would not be considered the most beautiful physically, but they are decisively attractive in their own right. All of the above have had an enormous influence on many lives. They possess something special that, while hard to pin down, is very real. And while it's easy to point to someone's stunning qualities and say that basic beauty is the most important ingredient in star quality or popular appeal that would be just as wrong as saying that raw intelligence is the only aspect of being smart. Raw physical beauty, like intelligence and creative talent, is just one of the building blocks to being recognized as attractive. As we've seen throughout this book, the power of attraction involves much more.

> Bottom line, our innate desire to be beautiful is hardwired and evolutionarily motivated.

Our evolutionarily designed primitive minds are wired to perceive beauty as the most tangible and overt trait that defines someone as a carrier of good genes, and it is the oldest, most developed and best preserved function of beauty throughout the animal kingdom. Regardless of species, many animals flaunt their level of attractiveness to be more alluring to the opposite sex. From the simplest fish, reptiles, birds, and mammals, all the way up the evolutionary chain to humans, we try to showcase our talents to potential mates as well as our competitors. The reindeer buck with the largest antlers, for example, is more desirable to does and struts them proudly (Markusson & Folstad, 1997); peacocks with long beautiful tails show off their bright feathers

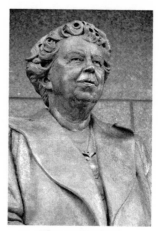

Eleanor Roosevelt

and have more mating success (Petrie, 1994); and male swordfish with longer swords are preferred by the ladies of the swordfish world (Basolo, 1990). Do you think things are much different for humans? It's natural to be motivated to exhibit our health and look great in order to help improve our level of attractiveness—this is consistent with our evolutionary predisposition.

However, unlike our evolutionary predecessors, humans have the ability to go well beyond our natural beauty to boost our attractiveness. From earliest recorded history we see that adornments such as piercings, lipstick, and hair dye have been used to highlight beauty and impress a would-be suitor. Remote tribal villages to this day still use the same tools as their ancestors did millennia ago to draw attention to their beauty, thereby increasing their levels of attractiveness. Even in times of famine, women have devoted resources to enhancing their appearance. These flattering behaviors are cross-cultural and consistent across civilizations and time periods.

> Humans have the ability to go well beyond our natural beauty to boost our attractiveness.

In the modern world, clothing styles, jewelry, makeup, hairstyles, facial hair on men, and yes, even morphologically altering cosmetic surgery, are options for highlighting and accentuating particular features of beauty in an attempt to be more attractive. Bottom line, our innate desire to be beautiful is hardwired and evolutionarily motivated. Those quick to denigrate having cosmetic treatments as a vain, unnatural self-obsession are really denying the basic human urge to want to look better and increase their level of attractiveness, which has proven to make a significant positive difference in every aspect of life.

In modern society, the term "vanity" translates as excessive pride in one's appearance and being conceited, overly self-centered and narcissistic in looks and attitude. From my view, this is unfair, because I've seen first-hand how even the most minor cosmetic alterations can enhance self-esteem and start the domino effect of a better life. Being vain enough to care about one's self and image is essential to being attractive and human.

Attractiveness is a dynamic, multifaceted and visceral calling that helps facilitate our only evolutionary goal—both individually and collectively as a species—the survival of our genes. It's important to keep in mind that in the more evolutionarily advanced species, beauty is but one component of being attractive. While beauty may

> First impressions are based on how you feel as much as on how you look.

have a disproportionate influence on attractiveness, it alone does not equal attraction. Those who seek out adornments or plastic surgery with the hope that this alone will make them more attractive are wrong and misguided. As illustrated consistently throughout this book, being objectively beautiful is far different from being attractive.

The #1 Ingredient to Being Attractive and Enjoying Its Advantages

The plain hard truth is that how we look does matter—but only to a point. I would argue that in our modern and evolutionarily advanced species, our self-esteem and how that self-esteem is perceived are far more integral and influential components to attractiveness than physical beauty. You can be asymmetric with small, beady eyes, and thinning hair, but if your self-esteem is high, you will overcome the disadvantages that may be associated

In cosmetic medicine, my job is to alter brain chemistry by making people feel good about themselves, not necessarily by making them look better.

with those traits. People who perceive themselves as physically beautiful report that they have more satisfying social interactions, handle negative situations better, are more satisfied at work, and think they deserve more attractive mates (Garcia, Khersonsky & Stagey, 1997). On top of that, women with a higher self-perceived level of attractiveness are asked out on dates more often (Todd et al., 2007).

It all comes down to this: First impressions are based on how you feel as much as on how you look. When you feel good about yourself, you project yourself better. I say this with confidence, not only because I've seen for decades how this emotional link plays out in the higher quality of life of my patients, but also because science backs it up. For example, two recent studies show that one who internally feels more attractive is more apt to smile, and those who smile are rated nicer and friendlier by others. These scientists reported that "attraction is influenced not only by physical beauty, but also by the extent to which a person appears open to engaging the observer" (Jones, DeBruine, Little, Conway & Feinberg, 2006; Jones et al., 2005).

If you engage with someone warmly, affectionately and purposely, the other person recognizes this consciously and subconsciously. By talking to people you meet for the first time with purpose and even smiling at them, you not only increase how good they feel about themselves, but also positively alter how they perceive and treat you. There is a reason most United States presidents and legendary CEOs are said to be incredibly engaging and apt to make those around them feel better. The best of the best have mastered the art of being attractive and succeed by making those around them feel more attractive at the same time. This quality works because it's authentic: putting on a friendly face without feeling genuinely interested isn't the point. Mastering the art of attraction is about mastering traits of caring, respecting and being curious about people.

In cosmetic medicine, my job is to alter brain chemistry by making people feel good about themselves, not necessarily by making them look better. I think this point is important and deserves reiteration. As a plastic surgeon I don't make people look better, I make them feel better. This may sound counterintuitive, and is the reason my teaching and writing is often met with friction. Can you imagine telling a room full of doctors who have spent over a third of their life devoted to learning intricate anatomy, specialized surgical skills, and exquisite hand-eye coordination that they should shelve their technical aptitude from time to time and replace it with their social and listening skills instead? In my field, this approach is controversial, to say the least. It goes against the grain to profess that the goal of cosmetic medicine is not always to focus on ironing out a wrinkle, filling in a fold, or plumping a lip, but rather sometimes to have a conversation.

Although it varies for each person, up to seventy percent of our variance in self-esteem is wrapped up in feelings about our own physical attractiveness (Harter, 1993). For those who benefit, cosmetic interventions likely lead to alterations in levels of the feel-good brain chemicals serotonin and dopamine, which affect our quality of life and self-confidence. There are many ways to improve our disposition, and not all of them involve our appearance. Some people turn to drugs, alcohol or caffeine for a temporary improvement in their mood or attitude, regardless of whether or not they realize that using drugs or alcohol can lead to irresponsible actions, cause irreparable damage and bring you back to square one when they wear off. Others seek out the guidance of a professional counselor or coach to learn tools for building confidence. Another popular technique for invigorating self-esteem is through regular exercise or a loving relationship. Still others may enhance their self-esteem by excelling at school or working or serving others. Regardless of the tactic used to enhance self-esteem, the result is the same—increased attractiveness, both as perceived internally and as projected to others.

> Regardless of the tactic used to enhance self-esteem, the result is the same—increased attractiveness, both as perceived internally and as projected to others.

Fatal Extremes: Cockiness and Low Self-Esteem

Being down on yourself seems to make everything worse.

People with low self-esteem are hampered by feelings of being less likable, have a more negative response to unpleasant social interactions, report more stressful life events, and provide less social support than people with high self-esteem (Buhrmester, Furman, Wittenberg & Reis, 1988; Lakey, Tardiff & Drew, 1994). Unfortunately, one of the most consistent predictors of low self-esteem in women is a husband who criticizes or insults her appearance. For a man, lowered self-esteem often comes from a failure to achieve the expected amount of resources, such as money or social status as compared to those within their peer group.

> A healthy dose of self-esteem is strongly linked to having a greater resistance to depression, being better able to cope with life's stresses, and just being happier overall.

However, on the other end of the spectrum, too much self-esteem is not healthy or beneficial, either. Those who are grandiose or narcissistic tend to go from positive initial peer ratings to negative scores over time (Paulhus, 1998). Think of the cocky new guy at work who seems unique and exciting at first, but then starts to wear on people until he's considered nothing more than a self-absorbed blowhard. Too much self-esteem can be destructive, alienating, and lead to being disliked. At its worst, too much self-esteem morphs into the narcissism that leads to destroyed relationships, criminal behavior, and wars.

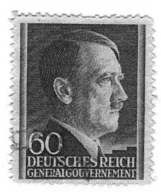

Hitler the ultimate narcissist.

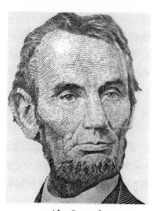

*Abe Lincoln
the ultimate leader.*

For the ninety-nine percent of the population that does not tip over into a narcissistic personality disorder, an elevated healthy dose of self-esteem is strongly linked to having a greater resistance to depression, being better able to cope with life's stresses, and just being happier overall. As obvious as it may sound, happiness is worth developing: it promotes success at work, personal autonomy, satisfaction with jobs, better performance on work-related tasks, and the likeliness of earning greater wealth across your lifetime (Boehm & Lyubomirsky, 2008).

Self-esteem seasoned with an altruistic concern for others—*benevolent self-esteem,* as I call it—is found in people who possess the confidence and resolve to help others, from a family member or neighbor to a suffering person a world away. Benevolent self-esteem is a character ingredient for the genius that starts industries, ends wars, influences friends, and changes the world.

Changing the World

Benevolent self-esteem is the highly elusive and treasured Holy Grail behind every lasting success, whether that is in parenting your children, leading the local PTA, being a Hollywood headliner or respected world leader. Developing your capacity for benevolent self-esteem opens up opportunities for controlling your own destiny and reaping all the benefits and advantages that come with it—for all of us.

Far from narcissistic or egotistical, benevolent self-esteem is a radical approach to changing yourself and the world.

Every chapter in this book has revealed insights into the designs and blueprints that define self-esteem and attractiveness. But to visualize and put them into motion requires thinking at the intersection where science, art, and humanism cross paths. It is here where all the lines and colors line up and a once-hazy outlook about life's purpose becomes clear. This is where the greats who change the world for the better, both for themselves and the rest of us, live. To grasp and live by a level of attraction that sets you up to achieve your highest potential and bring out the best in others, however, requires opening your

> Benevolent self-esteem is a character ingredient for the genius that starts industries, ends wars, influences friends, and changes the world.

mind and closely examining preconceived notions that come from religious, political or social doctrines. Once this path is visualized, the path to being attractive—in every sense of the word—will become obvious and you'll have a difficult time believing that at one time you didn't see it. It may be difficult for you to explain it to others because, much like the challenge of seeing those 3-D photos hiding within a random pattern, some people are too invested in their traditional filters to see another way.

> Benevolent self-esteem is the highly elusive and treasured Holy Grail behind every lasting success.

Like anything else you've learned, after a while your new approach to forming a strong and positive first impression becomes normal, you master another set of skills, your attractiveness increases, and you become a highly desirable and influential individual. As difficulties in your life arise, as they always will, the pits will be shallower, the hills smaller and distances shorter. Benevolent self-esteem blunts intimidation, squashes boredom, and brings purpose to all aspects of your life. It is the fuel that allows a mother and father to raise their children through the torrential storms of childhood and empowers leaders to persist in the face of obstacles and criticism.

> Forming a strong and positive first impression transforms you into a highly desirable and influential individual.

I hope that this journey through professional experiences, life lessons, art, and science has given you a solid grounding in the facts about beauty and attractiveness. Now that we've proven why we see people and act upon our most primitive drives and perceptions as we do, we can look at our lives and those we love from a much broader perspective. We know that people with high self-esteem are perceived by others to carry good genes, and this translates into an attractive image that over millions of years has fit in harmoniously within the evolutionary designs of Mother Nature, or whomever you would like to name the source of these plans. And while raw beauty is an important aspect of being attractive, irresistible people owe their powers of attraction to much more than the physical.

Being attractive is a state of mind, and like any other worthwhile possession, achieving it will not come easy. To get there requires mastering a new way of thinking, which demands hard work, practice, and failure before it becomes second nature. However, once you embrace this thinking you will always know how to make a better first impression, regardless of time, place, or circumstance. You will be able to count yourself among the enlightened few who have the skills and abilities to not only elevate themselves, but also all those around them. They truly are the beautiful.

Are you ready to be one of them?

"Where there is passion doubt cannot be."
—Steven H. Dayan

ACKNOWLEDGEMENTS:

To my friends, patients, staff, colleagues, teachers, students and especially my family, I owe everything. We exist as a mosaic of living experiences, collective, dynamic and heritable. I appreciate those who have instilled within me the ability to observe, listen and absorb and to those who granted me the privilege to influence. Whatever value that passes through me is nothing more than a confluence of their purpose and my attempt to interpret the meaning.

Thank you to Antonia Felix for her editorial support.

ABOUT THE AUTHOR

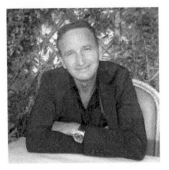

Steven Dayan, a born and raised Chicagoan, is an internationally renowned Board Certified Facial Plastic Surgeon, a frequent lecturer, physician educator and an active researcher in emerging cosmetic medicine technologies and techniques. He has published over 80 articles in medical journals and authored four books. As a clinical assistant professor at the University of Illinois he has trained 1000's of physicians worldwide. Over the years, Dr. Dayan has racked up a long list of professional accolades, including the American Medical Association (AMA) Foundation's Leadership Award and the Chicago Medical Society's Public Service Award. He has also been recognized as a "Top Doc" by numerous organizations including, Castle Connolly, U.S News and Report and Consumer Check Book Guides.

But it is in his role as an adjunct professor at DePaul University where he passionately teaches a wildly popular undergraduate course: *The Science of Beauty and Attraction and its Impact on Culture and Business* – that this book is based. A big thinker with an insatiable appetite for deeper knowledge and understanding of human behavior, Dr. Dayan is known for his ability to challenge the status quo of his students and the conventional wisdoms of modern medicine.

It's all part and parcel of his overall mission to empower individuals, businesses and societies to better understand the how and why behind their thoughts attitudes and actions.

REFERENCES

Abelove, H. (2005). *Deep Gossip*: University of Minnesota Press.

Alegria, C. A., & University of Nevada, R. S. P. (2008). *Relational maintenance and schema renegotiation following disclosure of transsexualism: An examination of sustaining male—to-female transsexual and natal female couples*: University of Nevada, Reno.

Aloha, A. S. (2010). Is Justice Really Blind? : Effects of Crime Descriptions, Defendant Gender and Appearance, and Legal Practitioner Gender on Sentences and Defendant Evaluations in a Mock Trial. *Psychiatry, Psychology and Law*(17), 304-324.

The American Society of Aesthetic Plastic Surgery. 2010 Statistics from The American Society of Aesthetic Plastic Surgery. (2011) Retrieved April 26, 2011, from http://www.surgery.org/sites/default/files/Stats2010_1.pdf

Anderson, J. L., Crawford, C. B., Nadeau, J., & Lindberg, T. (1992). Was the Duchess of windsor right? A cross-cultural review of the socioecology of ideals of female body shape. *Ethology and Sociobiology, 13*(3), 197-227. doi: 10.1016/0162-3095(92)90033-z

Axelsson, J., Sundelin, T., Ingre, M., Van Someren, E. J., Olsson, A., & Lekander, M. (2010). Beauty sleep: experimental study on the perceived health and attractiveness of sleep deprived people. *BMJ, 341*, c6614.

Bailey, C. M. (April 10, 2010). The evolution of dating: Match.com and Chadwick Martin Bailey Behavioral Studies uncover a fundamental shift., from http://blog.cmbinfo.com/press-center-content/bid/46915/The-Evolution-of-Dating-Match-com-and-Chadwick-Martin-Bailey-Behavioral-Studies-Uncover-a-Fundamental-Shift

Bailey, J. M., & Pillard, R. C. (1991). A Genetic Study of Male Sexual Orientation. *Arch Gen Psychiatry, 48*(12), 1089-1096. doi: 10.1001/archpsyc.1991.01810360053008

Baker, M. J., & Churchill, G. A. (1977). The impact of physically attractive models on advertising evaluations. *Journal of Marketing Research, 14*(4), 538-555. doi: 10.2307/3151194

Baker, R. R., & Bellis, M. A. (1995). *Human Sperm Competition: Copulation, Masturbation and Infidelity.* London: Chapman and Hall.

Basolo, A. L. (1990). Female preference for male sword length in the green swordtail, Xiphophorus helleri (Pisces: Poeciliidae). *Animal Behaviour, 40*(2), 332-338. doi: 10.1016/s0003-3472(05)80928-5

Baumeister, R. F., Campbell, J. D., Krueger, J. I., & Vohs, K. D. (2003). Does high self-esteem cause better performance, interpersonal success, happiness, or healthier lifestyles? *Psychological Science in the Public Interest, 4*(1), 1-44. doi: 10.1111/1529-1006.01431

Bellis, M. A., & Baker, R. R. (1990). Do females promote sperm competition? Data for humans. *Anim Behav, 40*, 997-990.

Bereczkei, T., & Csanaky, A. (1996). Mate choice, marital success, and reproduction in a modern society. *Ethol Sociobiol, 17*, 17-35.

Biddle, J. E., & Hamermesh, D. S. (1998). Beauty, Productivity, and Discrimination: Lawyers' Looks and Lucre. [Article]. *Journal of Labor Economics, 16*(1), 172.

Birmingham, C. L., Su, J., Hlynsky, J. A., Goldner, E. M., & Gao, M. (2005). The mortality rate from anorexia nervosa. *Int J Eat Disord, 38*(2), 143-146. doi: 10.1002/eat.20164

Blackwood, E. (1986). Breaking the mirror: The construction of lesbianism and the anthropoligcal discourse on homosexuality. In E. Blackwood (Ed.), *Anthropology and homosexual behaviour* (pp. 1-17). New York: Hawworth Press.

Blanchard, R., & Bogaert, A. (1996). Biodemographic comparisons of homosexual and heterosexual men in the kinsey interview data. *Archives of Sexual Behavior, 25*(6), 551-579. doi: 10.1007/bf02437839

Blanchard, R., & Bogaert, A. (1996). Homosexuality in men and number of older brothers. *Am J Psychiatry, 153*(1), 27-31.

Bloom, V., Niles, R., & Tatcher, A. (1995). Sources of marital dissatisfaction among newly separated persons. *J Fam Issues, 6*, 359-373.

Boehm, J. K., & Lyubomirsky, S. (2008). Does Happiness Promote Career Success? *Journal of Career Assessment, 16*(1), 101-116. doi: 10.1177/1069072707308140

Bonanno, G. A., Field, N. P., Kovacevic, A., & Kaltman, S. (2002). Self-Enhancement as a Buffer Against Extreme Adversity: Civil War in Bosnia and Traumatic Loss in the United States. *Personality and Social Psychology Bulletin, 28*(2), 184-196. doi: 10.1177/0146167202282005

Booth, A., & Edwards, J. (1985). Age at marriage and marriage instability. *J Marriage Fam, 47*, 67-75.

Buhrmester, D., Furman, W., Wittenberg, M. T., & Reis, H. T. (1988). Five domains of interpersonal competence in peer relationships. *Journal of Personality and Social Psychology, 55*(6), 991-1008. doi: 10.1037/0022-3514.55.6.991

Bulpitt, C. J., Markowe, H. L., & Shipley, M. J. (2001). Why do some people look older than they should? *Postgrad Med J, 77*(911), 578-581.

Burkett, L. (1989). *Debt-Free Living: How to Get Out of Debt (and Stay Out)*. Chicago, IL: Moody Press.

Burnham, T. C., Chapman, J. F., Gray, P. B., McIntyre, M. H., Lipson, S. F., & Ellison, P. T. (2003). Men in committed, romantic relationships have lower testosterone. *Horm Behav, 44*(2), 119-122.

Buss, D. M. (1989). *Sex differences in human mate preferences: evolutionary hypotheses tested in 37 cultures* (Vol. 12). Cambridge, ROYAUME-UNI: Cambridge University Press.

Buss, D. M. (1994/2003). *The Evolution of Desire: Strategies of Human Mating*. New York: Basic Books.

Buss, D. M. (2004). *Evolutionary Psychology: The New Science of the Mind* (2 ed.). Boston: Allyn and Bacon.

Buss, D. M., Larsen, R. J., Westen, D., & Semmelroth, J. (1992). Sex differences in jealousy: Evolution, physiology, and psychology. *Psych Sci, 3*, 251-255.

Buss, D. M., & Schmitt, D. P. (1993). Sexual strategies theory: an evolutionary perspective on human mating. *Psychol Rev, 100*(2), 204-232.

Buss, D. M., Shackelford, T. K., & LeBlanc, G. J. (2000). Number of children desired and preferred spousal age difference: context-specific mate preference patterns across 37 cultures. *Evol Hum Behav, 21*(5), 323-331.

Cárdenas, R. A., & Harris, L. J. (2006). Symmetrical decorations enhance the attractiveness of faces and abstract designs. *Evolution and Human Behavior, 27*(1), 1-18. doi: 10.1016/j.evolhumbehav.2005.05.002

Carré, J. M., & McCormick, C. M. (2008). In your face: Facial metrics predict aggressive behaviour in the laboratory and in varsity and professional hockey players. *Proc Biol Sci, 275*(1651), 2651-2656.

Carrington, M., Nelson, G. W., Martin, M. P., Kissner, T., Vlahov, D., Goedert, J. J., . . . O'Brien, S. J. (1999). HLA and HIV-1: heterozygote advantage and B*35-Cw*04 disadvantage. *Science, 283*(5408), 1748-1752.

Cerda-Flores, R. M., Barton, S. A., Marty-Gonzalez, L. F., Rivas, F., & Chakraborty, R. (1999). Estimation of nonpaternity in the Mexican population of Nuevo Leon: a validation study with blood group markers. *Am J Phys Anthropol, 109*(3), 281-293.

Cesarini, J. P., Michel, L., Maurette, J. M., Adhoute, H., & Bejot, M. (2003). Immediate effects of UV radiation on the skin: modification by an antioxidant complex containing carotenoids. *Photodermatol Photoimmunol Photomed, 19*(4), 182-189. doi: 044 [pii]

Christensen, K., Iachina, M., Rexbye, H., Tomassini, C., Frederiksen, H., McGue, M., & Vaupel, J. W. (2004). "Looking old for your age": genetics and mortality. *Epidemiology, 15*(2), 251-252.

Chung, K. C., Hamill, J. B., Kim, H. M., Walters, M. R., & Wilkins, E. G. (1999). Predictors of patient satisfaction in an outpatient plastic surgery clinic. *Ann Plast Surg, 42*(1), 56-60.

Clark, R. D., & Hatfield, E. (1989). Gender differences in receptivity to sexual offers. *J Psych Hum Sex, 2*, 39-55.

Clayson, D., & Maughn, M. (1976). Paper presented at the Rocky Mountain Psychological Association, Phoenix AZ.

Clements-Nolle, K., Marx, R., Guzman, R., & Katz, M. (2001). HIV prevalence, risk behaviors, health care use, and mental health status of transgender persons: implications for public health intervention. *Am J Public Health, 91*(6), 915-921.

Clements-Nolle, K., Marx, R., & Katz, M. (2006). Attempted Suicide Among Transgender Persons: The Influence of Gender-Based Discrimination and Victimization. *Journal of Homosexuality, 51*(3), 53-69. doi: 10.1300/J082v51n03_04

Collins, M. A., & Zebrowitz, L. A. (1995). The Contributions of Appearance to Occupational Outcomes in Civilian and Military Settings1. *Journal of Applied Social Psychology, 25*(2), 129-163. doi: 10.1111/j.1559-1816.1995.tb01588.x

Committee, I. o. M. o. t. N. A. (2006). Progress in Preventing Childhood Obesity: How Do We Measure Up?

Corson, R. (1972). *Fashions in makeup, from ancient to modern times.* London,: Owen.

Cosmides, L., & Tooby, J. (1994). Origins of domain-specificity: The evolution of functional organization. In Hirschfeld LA & Gelman SA (Eds.), *Mapping the Mind: Domain Specificity in Cognition and Culture* (pp. 163-228). New York, NY: Oxford University Press.

Cunningham, M. R., Roberts, A. R., Barbee, A. P., Druen, P. B., & Wu, C.-H. (1995). "Their ideas of beauty are, on the whole, the same as ours": Consistency and variability in the cross-cultural perception of female physical attractiveness. *Journal of Personality and Social Psychology, 68*(2), 261-279. doi: 10.1037/0022-3514.68.2.261

Currie, T. E., & Little, A. C. (2009). The relative importance of the face and body in judgments of human physical attractiveness. *Evol Hum Behav, 30*, 409-416.

Dabbs, J. M., Jurkovic, G. J., & Frady, R. L. (1991). Salivary testosterone and cortisol among late adolescent male offenders. *Journal of Abnormal Child Psychology, 19*(4), 469-478. doi: 10.1007/bf00919089

Darr, D., Combs, S., Dunston, S., Manning, T., & Pinnell, S. (1992). Topical vitamin C protects porcine skin from ultraviolet radiation-induced damage. *Br J Dermatol, 127*(3), 247-253.

Darr, D., Dunston, S., Faust, H., & Pinnell, S. (1996). Effectiveness of antioxidants (vitamin C and E) with and without sunscreens as topical photoprotectants. *Acta Derm Venereol, 76*(4), 264-268.

Dayan, S., Clark, K., & Ho, A. A. (2004). Altering first impressions after facial plastic surgery. *Aesthetic Plast Surg, 28*(5), 301-306. doi: 10.1007/s00266-004-1017-1

Dayan, S. H., Arkins, J. P., & Gal, T. J. (2010). Blinded evaluation of the effects of hyaluronic acid filler injections on first impressions. *Dermatol Surg, 36 Suppl 3*, 1866-1873. doi: 10.1111/j.1524-4725.2010.01737.x

Dayan, S. H., Arkins, J. P., & Mussman, C. (2011). Looking in the Mirror: An Evaluation of Vanity in Patients Receiving Botulinum Toxin Treatments. *Cosmetic Dermatology, 24*(6), 263-266.

Dayan, S. H., Arkins, J. P., Patel, A. B., & Gal, T. J. (2010). A Double-Blind, Randomized, Placebo-Controlled Health-Outcomes Survey of the Effect of Botulinum Toxin Type A Injections on Quality of Life and Self-Esteem. *Dermatologic Surgery, 36*, 2088-2097. doi: 10.1111/j.1524-4725.2010.01795.x

Dayan, S. H., Lieberman, E. D., Thakkar, N. N., Larimer, K. A., & Anstead, A. (2008). Botulinum toxin a can positively impact first impression. *Dermatol Surg, 34 Suppl 1*, S40-47. doi: DSU34241 [pii]
10.1111/j.1524-4725.2008.34241.x

De Block, A., & Adriaens, P. (2004). Darwinizing sexual ambivalence: a new evolutionary hypothesis of male homosexuality. *Philosophical Psychology, 17*(1), 59-76. doi: 10.1080/0951508042000202381

Dean, T., & Lane, C. (2001). *Homosexuality & psychoanalysis*: University of Chicago Press.

Diener, E., Wolsic, B., & Fujita, F. (1995). Physical Attractiveness and Subjective Well-Being. *Journal of Personality and Social Psychology, 69*(1), 120-129.

Diffey, B. L. (2002). Human exposure to solar ultraviolet radiation. *J Cosmet Dermatol, 1*(3), 124-130. doi: JCD060 [pii]
10.1046/j.1473-2165.2002.00060.x

Dixson, B. J., Dixson, A. F., Li, B., & Anderson, M. J. (2007). Studies of human physique and sexual attractiveness: sexual preferences of men and women in China. *Am J Hum Biol, 19*(1), 88-95.

Dixson, B. J., Grimshaw, G. M., Linklater, W. L., & Dixson, A. F. (2011). Eye-tracking of men's preferences for waist-to-hip ratio and breast size of women. *Arch Sex Behav, 40*(1), 43-50.

Dnes, A. W., & Rowthorn, R. (2002). *The Law and Economics of Marriage and Divorce*. Cambridge: Cambridge University Press.

Draelos, Z. D. (2005). *Cosmeceuticals*: Elsevier Saunders.

Ekman, P. (1982). Does the face provide accurate information? . In P. Ekman (Ed.), *Emotion the Human Face* (2nd ed., pp. 56-97). Cambridge, England: Cambridge University Press.

Ermisch, J. (1993). Familia oeconomica: A survey of the economics of the family. *Scott J Pol Econ, 40,* 353-374.

Ertem, M., & Kocturk, T. (2008). Opinions on early-age marriage and marriage customs among Kurdish-speaking women in southeast Turkey. *J Fam Plann Reprod Health Care, 34*(3), 147-152.

Etcoff, N. (2000). *Survival of the prettiest: the science of beauty*: Anchor Books.

Etcoff, N., Orbach, S., Scott, J., & H., D. A. (2006). "Beyond Stereotypes: Rebuilding the Foundation of Beauty Beliefs":

Findings of the 2005 Dove Global Study: Dove, a Unilever Beauty Brand.

Evans, L., Kennedy, G. A., & Wertheim, E. H. (2005). An examination of the association between eating problems, negative mood, weight and sleeping quality in young women and men. *Eat Weight Disord, 10*(4), 245-250.

Ewing, D. J., Neilson, J. M., Shapiro, C. M., Stewart, J. A., & Reid, W. (1991). Twenty four hour heart rate variability: effects of posture, sleep, and time of day in healthy controls and comparison with bedside tests of autonomic function in diabetic patients. *British Heart Journal, 65*(5), 239-244. doi: 10.1136/hrt.65.5.239

Farkas, L. G., & Cheung, G. (1981). Facial asymmetry in healthy North American Caucasians. An anthropometrical study. *Angle Orthod, 51*(1), 70-77.

Fay, R., Turner, C., Klassen, A., & Gagnon, J. (1989). Prevalence and patterns of same-gender sexual contact among men. *Science, 243*(4889), 338-348. doi: 10.1126/science.2911744

Ferrucci, L., Cherubini, A., Bandinelli, S., Bartali, B., Corsi, A., Lauretani, F., . . . Guralnik, J. M. (2006). Relationship of plasma polyunsaturated fatty acids to circulating inflammatory markers. *J Clin Endocrinol Metab, 91*(2), 439-446. doi: 10.1210/jc.2005-1303

Fink, B., Neave, N., & Seydel, H. (2007). Male facial appearance signals physical strength to women. *Am J Hum Biol, 19*(1), 82-87. doi: 10.1002/ajhb.20583

Fitzpatrick, K. K., Euton, S. J., Jones, J. N., & Schmidt, N. B. (2005). Gender role, sexual orientation and suicide risk. *Journal of Affective Disorders, 87*(1), 35-42. doi: 10.1016/j.jad.2005.02.020

Fournier, P. F. (2002). The Lorenz theory of beauty. *Journal of Cosmetic Dermatology, 1*(3), 131-136. doi: 10.1046/j.1473-2165.2002.00038.x

Foustanos, A., Pantazi, L., & Zavrides, H. (2007). Representations in Plastic Surgery: The Impact of Self-Image and Self-Confidence in the Work Environment. *Aesthetic Plastic Surgery, 31*(5), 435-442. doi: 10.1007/s00266-006-0070-3

Francken, A. B., van de Wiel, H. B., van Driel, M. F., & Weijmar Schultz, W. C. (2002). What importance do women attribute to the size of the penis? *Eur Urol, 42*(5), 426-431.

Freeman, J. B., Johnson, K. L., Ambady, N., & Rule, N. O. (2010). Sexual Orientation Perception Involves Gendered Facial Cues. *Personality and Social Psychology Bulletin, 36*(10), 1318-1331. doi: 10.1177/0146167210378755

Frieze, I. H., Olson, J. E., & Good, D. C. (1990). Perceived and actual discrimination in the salaries of male and female managers. *J Applied Social Psych, 20*, 46-47.

Furnham, A., & Baguma, P. (1994). Cross-cultural differences in the evaluation of male and female body shapes. *International Journal of Eating Disorders, 15*(1), 81-89. doi: 10.1002/1098-108x(199401)15:1<81::aid-eat2260150110>3.0.co;2-d

Gallup, G. G., Burch, R. L., Zappieri, M. L., Parvez, R., Stockwell, M., & Davis, J. A. (2003). The human penis as a semen displacement device. *Evol Hum Behav, 24*, 277-289.

Gangestad, S. W., & Buss, D. M. (1993). Pathogen prevalence and human mate preferences. *Ethology and Sociobiology, 14*(2), 89-96. doi: 10.1016/0162-3095(93)90009-7

Gangestad, S. W., & Cousins, A. J. (2001). Adaptive design, female mate preferences, and shifts across the menstrual cycle. *Annu Rev Sex Res, 12*, 145-185.

Gangestad, S. W., Simpson, J. A., Cousins, A. J., Garver-Apgar, C. E., & Christensen, P. N. (2004). Women's preferences for male behavioral displays change across the menstrual cycle. *Psychol Sci, 15*(3), 203-207.

Gangestad, S. W., & Thornhill, R. (1998). Menstrual cycle variation in women's preferences for the scent of symmetrical men. *Proc Biol Sci, 265*(1399), 927-933.

Gangestad, S. W., Thornhill, R., & Garver, C. E. (2002). Changes in women's sexual interests and their partners' mate-retention tactics across the menstrual cycle: evidence for shifting conflicts of interest. *Proc Biol Sci, 269*(1494), 975-982.

Garcia, S. D., Khersonsky, D., & Stagey, S. (1997). Self-Perceptions of Physical Attractiveness. *Perceptual and Motor Skills, 84*(1), 243-250. doi: 10.2466/pms.1997.84.1.243

Garner, D. (1997). Survey says: Body image poll results. *Psychology Today, 30*(1).

Garver-Apgar, C. E., Gangestad, S. W., Thornhill, R., Miller, R. D., & Olp, J. J. (2006). Major histocompatibility complex alleles, sexual responsivity, and unfaithfulness in romantic couples. *Psychol Sci, 17*(10), 830-835.

Gaunt, R. (2006). Couple similarity and marital satisfaction: are similar spouses happier? *J Pers, 74*(5), 1401-1420.

Geiselman, R. E., Haight, N. A., & Kimata, L. G. (1984). Context effects on the perceived physical attractiveness of faces. *Journal of Experimental Social Psychology, 20*(5), 409-424. doi: 10.1016/0022-1031(84)90035-0

Gensler, H. L., & Magdaleno, M. (1991). Topical vitamin E inhibition of immunosuppression and tumorigenesis induced by ultraviolet irradiation. *Nutr Cancer, 15*(2), 97-106.

Getz, J. G., & Klein, H. K. (1980). *The frosting of the American woman: hairdressing and the phenomenology of beauty.* Paper presented at the Society for the Study of Social Problems, New York.

Gladwell, M. (2005). *Blink: the power of thinking without thinking.* Little, Brown and Co.

Global Industry Analysts, I. (February 2011). Fragrance and Perfumes Market Report.

Graham, J. A., & Jouhar, A. J. (1981). The effects of cosmetics on person perception. *International Journal of Cosmetic Science, 3*(5), 199-210. doi: 10.1111/j.1467-2494.1981.tb00283.x

Grammer, K., Fink, B., Moller, A. P., & Thornhill, R. (2003). Darwinian aesthetics: sexual selection and the biology of beauty. *Biol Rev Camb Philos Soc, 78*(3), 385-407.

Grammer, K., Fink, B., Møller, A. P., & Thornhill, R. (2003). Darwinian aesthetics: sexual selection and the biology of beauty. *Biol Rev Camb Philos Soc, 78*(3), 385-407.

Grammer, K., Fink, B., & Neave, N. (2005). Human pheromones and sexual attraction. *Eur J Obstet Gynecol Reprod Biol, 118*(2), 135-142.

Greenberg, D. F. (1988). *The consruction of homosexuality.* Chicago: University of Chicago Press.

Gunn, D. A., Rexbye, H., Griffiths, C. E., Murray, P. G., Fereday, A., Catt, S. D., ... Christensen, K. (2009). Why some women look young for their age. *PLoS One, 4*(12), e8021.

Hamermesh, D. (2006). Changing looks and changing "discrimination": The beauty of economists. *Econ Lett, 93,* 405-412.

Hamermesh, D., & Biddle, J. E. (1994). Beauty and the Labor Market. *The American Economic Review, 84*(5), 1174-1194.

Harris, M. B., Walters, L. C., & Waschull, S. (1991). Gender and ethnic differences in obesity-related behaviors and attitudes in a college sample. *J Applied Social Psych, 21,* 1545-1577.

Harter, S. (1993). Causes and consequences of low self-esteem in children and adolescents *Self-esteem: The puzzle of low self-regard.* (pp. 87-116): New York, NY, US: Plenum Press.

Haselton, M. G., & Buss, D. M. (2001). Emotional reactions following first-time sexual intercourse: The affective shift hypothesis. *Pers Rel, 8,* 357-369.

Haselton, M. G., Buss, D. M., Oubaid, V., & Angleitner, A. (2005). Sex, lies, and strategic interference: The psychology of deception between the sexes. *Pers Soc Psych Bull, 31*(1), 3-23.

Havlicek, J., Roberts, S. C., & Flegr, J. (2005). Women's preference for dominant male odour: effects of menstrual cycle and relationship status. *Biol Lett, 1*(3), 256-259.

Hendrickx, H., McEwen, B. S., & Ouderaa, F. v. d. (2005). Metabolism, mood and cognition in aging: The importance of lifestyle and dietary intervention. *Neurobiology of Aging, 26*(1, Supplement), 1-5. doi: 10.1016/j.neurobiolaging.2005.10.005

Hirsch, A. R. (1998). Scent and sexual arousal. *Med Aspects Hum Sexuality, 1*, 9-12.

Hirsch, A. R., Gruss, J., Bermele, C., Zagorski, D., & Schroder, M. A. (1998). The effects of odors on female sexual arousal. *Psychosomatic Med, 60*, 95.

Hirsch, R. J., Cohen, J. L., & Carruthers, J. D. (2007). Successful management of an unusual presentation of impending necrosis following a hyaluronic acid injection embolus and a proposed algorithm for management with hyaluronidase. *Dermatol Surg, 33*(3), 357-360. doi: 10.1111/j.1524-4725.2007.33073.x

Holme, S. A., Beattie, P. E., & Fleming, C. J. (2002). Cosmetic camouflage advice improves quality of life. *British Journal of Dermatology, 147*(5), 946-949. doi: 10.1046/j.1365-2133.2002.04900.x

Horn, J. C. (1979). Is it true Blonds seem less dumb? *Psychology Today*(October: 116).

Houser, M., Horan, S., & Furler, L. (2007). Predicting relational outcomes: An investigation of thin slice judgments in speed dating. *Hum Comm, 10*, 69-81.

Jacob, S., McClintock, M. K., Zelano, B., & Ober, C. (2002). Paternally inherited HLA alleles are associated with women's choice of male odor. *Nat Genet, 30*(2), 175-179.

Jansen, J. (December 30, 2010). Cash for content. Pew Internet & American Life Project, from http://pewresearch.org/pubs/1842/internet-users-pay-download-access-online-content

Janus, S., & Janus, C. L. (1993). *The Janus report on sexual behavior*: Wiley.

Jasienska, G., Ziomkiewicz, A., Ellison, P. T., Lipson, S. F., & Thune, I. (2004). Large breasts and narrow waists indicate high reproductive potential in women. *Proc Biol Sci, 271*(1545), 1213-1217. doi: 10.1098/rspb.2004.2712

Johnson, J. M. (1998). Physical training and the control of skin blood flow. *Medicine & Science in Sports & Exercise, 30*(3), 382-386.

Johnston, V. S., Hagel, R., Franklin, M., Fink, B., & Grammer, K. (2001). Male facial attractiveness: evidence for hormone-mediated adaptive design. *Evol Hum Behav, 22*, 251-267.

Johnston, V. S., Solomon, C. J., Gibson, S. J., & Pallares-Bejarano, A. (2003). Human facial beauty: current theories and methodologies. *Arch Facial Plast Surg, 5*(5), 371-377.

Jones, B. C., DeBruine, L. M., Little, A. C., Conway, C. A., & Feinberg, D. R. (2006). Integrating Gaze Direction and Expression in Preferences for Attractive Faces. *Psychological Science, 17*(7), 588-591. doi: 10.1111/j.1467-9280.2006.01749.x

Jones, B. C., Little, A. C., Boothroyd, L., Debruine, L. M., Feinberg, D. R., Smith, M. J., . . . Perrett, D. I. (2005). Commitment to relationships and preferences for femininity and apparent health in faces are strongest on days of the menstrual cycle when progesterone level is high. *Horm Behav, 48*(3), 283-290.

Jones, D. (2008). The bald truth about CEOs, *USA Today*.

Jones, D., & Hill, K. (1993). Criteria for facial attractiveness in five populations. *Human Nature, 4,* 271-295.

Jones, D., & Hill, K. (1993). Criteria of facial attractiveness in five populations. *Human Nature, 4*(3), 271-296. doi: 10.1007/bf02692202

Kaye, S. A., Folsom, A. R., Prineas, R. J., Potter, J. D., & Gapstur, S. M. (1990). The association of body fat distribution with lifestyle and reproductive factors in a population study of postmenopausal women. *Int J Obes, 14*(7), 583-591.

Kenagy, G. P. (2005). Transgender Health: Findings from Two Needs Assessment Studies in Philadelphia. *Health and Social Work, 30*(1), 19-26.

Kenrick, D. T., & Gutierres, S. E. (1980). Contrast effects and judgments of physical attractiveness: When beauty becomes a social problem. *Journal of Personality and Social Psychology, 38*(1), 131-140. doi: 10.1037/0022-3514.38.1.131

Kenrick, D. T., Gutierres, S. E., & Goldberg, L. L. (1989). Influence of popular erotica on judgments of strangers and mates. *Journal of Experimental Social Psychology, 25*(2), 159-167. doi: 10.1016/0022-1031(89)90010-3

Kenrick, D. T., Montello, D. R., Gutierres, S. E., & Trost, M. R. (1993). Effects of Physical Attractiveness on Affect and Perceptual Judgments: When Social Comparison Overrides Social Reinforcement. *Personality and Social Psychology Bulletin, 19*(2), 195-199. doi: 10.1177/0146167293192008

Kinsey, A. C., Pomeroy, W. B., & Martin, C. E. (2010). *Sexual behavior in the human male*. Bronx, N.Y.: Ishi Press Int.

Kirk-Smith, M. D., Booth, D. A., Carroll, D., & Davies, P. (1978). Human social attitudes affected by androstenol. *Res Commun Psychol Psychiatr Behav, 3*, 379-384.

Kowner, R., & Ogawa, T. (1993). The contrast effect of physical attractiveness in Japan. *J Psych, 127*, 51-64.

Koyama, N. F., McGain, A., & Hill, R. A. (2004). Self-reported mate preferences and"feminist"attitudes regarding marital relations. *Evol Hum Behav, 25*, 327-335.

Kruger, D. J., & Hughes, S. (2010). Variation in reproductive strategies influences post-coital experiences with partners. *J Soc Evol Cult Psych, 4*, 254-264.

Kruijver, F. P., Zhou, J. N., Pool, C. W., Hofman, M. A., Gooren, L. J., & Swaab, D. F. (2000). Male-to-female transsexuals have female neuron numbers in a limbic nucleus. *J Clin Endocrinol Metab, 85*(5), 2034-2041.

Laeng, B., & Falkenberg, L. (2007). Women's pupillary responses to sexually significant others during the hormonal cycle. *Horm Behav, 52*(4), 520-530.

Lakey, B., Tardiff, T. A., & Drew, J. B. (1994). Negative social interactions: Assessment and relations to social support, cognition, and psychological distress. *Journal of Social and Clinical Psychology, 13*(1), 42-62.

Landén, M., Wålinder, J., & Lundström, B. (1996). Prevalence, incidence and sex ratio of transsexualism. *Acta Psychiatrica Scandinavica, 93*(4), 221-223. doi: 10.1111/j.1600-0447.1996.tb10638.x

Langlois, J. H., & Roggman, L. (1990). Attractive faces are only average. *Psychol Science, 1*, 115-121.

Langlois, J. H., Roggman, L. A., Casey, R. J., Ritter, J. M., Rieser-Danner, L. A., & Jenkins, V. Y. (1987). Infant preferences for attractive faces: Rudiments of a stereotype? *Developmental Psychology, 23*(3), 363-363-369. doi: 10.1037/0012-1649.23.3.363

Langlois, J. H., Roggman, L. A., & Rieser-Danner, L. A. (1990). Infants' differential social responses to attractive and unattractive faces. *Developmental Psychology, 26*(1), 153-153-159. doi: 10.1037/0012-1649.26.1.153

Laser, P. S., & Mathie, V. A. (1982). Face facts: An unbidden role for features in communication. *Journal of Nonverbal Behavior, 7*(1), 3-19. doi: 10.1007/bf01001774

Laumann, A. E., & Derick, A. J. (2006). Tattoos and body piercings in the United States: a national data set. *J Am Acad Dermatol, 55*(3), 413-421. doi: 10.1016/j.jaad.2006.03.026

Levenson, R. W., Carstensen, L. L., & Gottman, J. M. (1993). Long-term marriage: Age, gender, and satisfaction. *Psychol Aging, 8*(2), 301-313.

Lever, J., Frederick, D. A., & Peplau, L. A. (2006). Does size matter? Men's and women's views on penis size across the lifespan. *Psych Men Masc, 7*, 129-143.

Lewis, M. B., & Bowler, P. J. (2009). Botulinum toxin cosmetic therapy correlates with a more positive mood. *J Cosmet Dermatol, 8*(1), 24-26. doi: 10.1111/j.1473-2165.2009.00419.x

Lindberg, L., & Hjern, A. (2003). Risk factors for anorexia nervosa: a national cohort study. *Int J Eat Disord, 34*(4), 397-408. doi: 10.1002/eat.10221

Little, A. C., Burriss, R. P., Jones, B. C., Debruine, L. M., & Caldwell, C. A. (2008). Social influence in human face preference: men and women are influenced more for long-term than short-term attractiveness decisions. *Evol Hum Behav, 29*, 140-146.

Little, A. C., Jones, B. C., Penton-Voak, I. S., Burt, D. M., & Perrett, D. I. (2002). Partnership status and the temporal context of relationships influence human female preferences for sexual dimorphism in male face shape. *Proc Biol Sci, 269*(1496), 1095-1100.

Lown, J. M., & Chandler, S. (1993). Financial problems as a contributing factor in divorce. *Proc Assoc Fin Coun Plan Ed*, 84-93.

Lyness, K. S., & Heilman, M. E. (2006). When fit is fundamental: Performance evaluations and promotions of upper-level female and male managers. *Journal of Applied Psychology, 91*(4), 777-785. doi: 10.1037/0021-9010.91.4.777

Lyness, K. S., & Thompson, D. E. (1997). Above the glass ceiling? A comparison of matched samples of female and male executives. *Journal of Applied Psychology, 82*(3), 359-375. doi: 10.1037/0021-9010.82.3.359

Malatesta, C. Z., Fiore, M. J., & Messina, J. J. (1987). Affect, personality, and facial expressive characteristics of older people. *Psychology and Aging, 2*(1), 64-69. doi: 10.1037/0882-7974.2.1.64

Markusson, E., & Folstad, I. (1997). Reindeer antlers: visual indicators of individual quality? *Oecologia, 110*(4), 501-507. doi: 10.1007/s004420050186

Masters, W., & Johnson, V. E. (2010). *Human Sexual Response*: Ishi Press International.

Masters, W. H., & Johnson, V. E. (2010). *Human Sexual Inadequacy*: Ishi Press International.

Mazur, A., & Booth, A. (1998). Testosterone and dominance in men. *Behav Brain Sci, 21*(3), 353-363.

Mazur, A., Mazur, J., & Keating, C. (1984). Military rank attainment of a West Point Class: Effects of cadet's physical features. *Am J of Sociology, 90*, 125-150.

McArdle, F., Rhodes, L. E., Parslew, R. A., Close, G. L., Jack, C. I., Friedmann, P. S., & Jackson, M. J. (2004). Effects of oral vitamin E and beta-carotene supplementation on ultraviolet radiation-induced oxidative stress in human skin. *Am J Clin Nutr, 80*(5), 1270-1275.

McAuley, E., Mihalko, S. L., & Bane, S. M. (1997). Exercise and self-esteem in middle-aged adults: multidimensional relationships and physical fitness and self-efficacy influences. *J Behav Med, 20*(1), 67-83.

McCarthy, E. (2009, Dec 20). Small lies about height or weight are frequently on online dating site profiles, *Washington Post*.

McClelland, E. E., Penn, D. J., & Potts, W. K. (2003). Major histocompatibility complex heterozygote superiority during coinfection. *Infect Immun, 71*(4), 2079-2086.

McNulty, J. K., Neff, L. A., & Karney, B. R. (2008). Beyond initial attraction: physical attractiveness in newlywed marriage. *J Fam Psychol, 22*(1), 135-143.

Meningaud, J.-P., Benadiba, L., Servant, J.-M., Herve, C., Bertrand, J.-C., & Pelicier, Y. (2003). Depression, anxiety and quality of life: outcome 9 months after facial cosmetic surgery. *Journal of Cranio-Maxillofacial Surgery, 31*(1), 46-50. doi: 10.1016/s1010-5182(02)00159-2

Metraux, A., & Kirchoff, P. (1948). The northeastern extension of Andean culture. In J. H. Steward (Ed.), *Handbook of South American Indians* (Vol. 4, pp. 349-368). Washington, D.C.: U.S. Government Printing OFfice.

Miller, G. (2008). Sexual Selection for Indicators of Intelligence *The Nature of Intelligence* (pp. 260-275): John Wiley & Sons, Ltd.

Montoya, R. M. (2008). I'm hot, so i'd say you're not: the influence of objective physical attractiveness on mate selection. *Pers Soc Psychol Bull, 34*(10), 1315-1331. doi: 0146167208320387 [pii] 10.1177/0146167208320387

Morgan, S. P., Lye, D. N., & Condran, G. A. (1988). Sons, daughters, and the risk of marital disruption. *Am J Sociol, 94*(1), 110-129.

Morris, D. (Writer) & D. Morris (Director). (1997). The Human Sexes. USA.

Mulford, M., Orbell, J., Shatto, C., & Stockard, J. (1998). *Physical attractiveness, opportunity, and success in everyday exchange* (Vol. 103). Chicago, IL, ETATS-UNIS: University of Chicago Press.

Muller, U., & Mazur, A. (1997). Facial dominance in Homo sapiens as honest signaling of male quality. *Behav Ecol, 8*, 569-579.

Murray, J. E. (2000). Marital protection and marital selection: Evidence from a historical-prospective sample of American men. *Demography, 37*(4), 511-521.

Nash, R., Fieldman, G., Hussey, T., Lévêque, J.-L., & Pineau, P. (2006). Cosmetics: They Influence More Than Caucasian Female Facial Attractiveness. *Journal of Applied Social Psychology, 36*(2), 493-504. doi: 10.1111/j.0021-9029.2006.00016.x

National Center on Sleep Disorders Research and Office of Prevention, E., and Control. (1997). Working Group Report on Problem Sleepiness: U.S. Department of Health and Human Services.

Naumann, L. P., Vazire, S., Rentfrow, P. J., & Gosling, S. D. (2009). Personality Judgments Based on Physical Appearance. *Personality and Social Psychology Bulletin, 35*(12), 1661-1671. doi: 10.1177/0146167209346309

Neave, N., Laing, S., Fink, B., & Manning, J. T. (2003). Second to fourth digit ratio, testosterone and perceived male dominance. *Proc Biol Sci, 270*(1529), 2167-2172.

Nelson, L. D., & Norton, M. I. (2005). From student to superhero: Situational primes shape finances impact preferences for potential partners. *Psych Science, 16*, 167-173.

Newell, R. (2000). Psychological difficulties amongst plastic surgery ex-patients following surgery tothe face: a survey. *British Journal of Plastic Surgery, 53*(5), 386-392. doi: 10.1054/bjps.1999.3273

Ober, C., Hyslop, T., Elias, S., Weitkamp, L. R., & Hauck, W. W. (1998). Human leukocyte antigen matching and fetal loss: results of a 10 year prospective study. *Hum Reprod, 13*(1), 33-38.

Ober, C. L., Hauck, W. W., Kostyu, D. D., E., O. B., Elias, S., Simpson, J. L., & Martin, A. O. (1985). Adverse effects of human leukocyte antigen-DR sharing on fertility: a cohort study in a human isolate. *Fertil Steril, 44*(2), 227-232.

Oberzaucher, E., & Grammer, K. (2009). Ageing, mate preferences and sexuality: a mini-review. *Gerontology, 55*(4), 371-378.

Oloruntoba-Oju, T. (2007). *Body Images, Beauty, Culture and Language in the Nigeria, African Context.* Paper presented at the Understanding Human Sexuality Seminar Series, University of Ibadan, Nigeria.

Olson, I. R., & Marshuetz, C. (2005). Facial Attractiveness Is Appraised in a Glance. *Emotion, 5*(4), 498-498-502. doi: 10.1037/1528-3542.5.4.498

Orange, R. (2011). Sperm bank turns down redheads, *The Telegraph.*

Parish, A. R. (1994). Sex and food control in the "uncommon chimanzee": How bonobo females overcome a phylogenetic legacy of male dominance. *Ethology and Sociobiology, 15*, 407-420.

Parker, G., Gibson, N. A., Brotchie, H., Heruc, G., Rees, A. M., & Hadzi-Pavlovic, D. (2006). Omega-3 fatty acids and mood disorders. *Am J Psychiatry, 163*(6), 969-978. doi: 10.1176/appi.ajp.163.6.969

Patel, S. R., Malhotra, A., White, D. P., Gottlieb, D. J., & Hu, F. B. (2006). Association between reduced sleep and weight gain in women. *Am J Epidemiol, 164*(10), 947-954. doi: 10.1093/aje/kwj280

Patzer, G. L. (1988). Psychologic and sociologic dimensions of hair: An aspect of the physical attractiveness phenomenon. *Clinics in Dermatology, 6*(4), 93-101. doi: 10.1016/0738-081x(88)90072-7

Paulhus, D. L. (1998). Interpersonal and intrapsychic adaptiveness of trait self-enhancement: A mixed blessing? *Journal of Personality and Social Psychology, 74*(5), 1197-1208. doi: 10.1037/0022-3514.74.5.1197

Pawlowski, B., & Sorokowski, P. (2008). Men's attraction to women's bodies changes seasonally. *Perception, 37*(7), 1079-1085.

Penton-Voak, I. S., Perrett, D. I., Castles, D. L., Kobayashi, T., Burt, D. M., Murray, L. K., & Minamisawa, R. (1999). Menstrual cycle alters face preference. *Nature, 399*(6738), 741-742.

Peplau, L., Frederick, D., Yee, C., Maisel, N., Lever, J., & Ghavami, N. (2009). Body Image Satisfaction in Heterosexual, Gay, and Lesbian Adults. *Archives of Sexual Behavior, 38*(5), 713-725. doi: 10.1007/s10508-008-9378-1

Petrie, M. (1994). Improved growth and survival of offspring of peacocks with more elaborate trains. [10.1038/371598a0]. *Nature, 371*(6498), 598-599.

Phillips, K. A., & Diaz, S. F. (1997). Gender Differences in Body Dysmorphic Disorder. *The Journal of Nervous and Mental Disease, 185*(9), 570-577.

Poduska, B., & Allred, G. H. (1990). Family finances: The missing link in MFT training. *Am J Fam Ther, 18*, 161-168.

Preti, G., Cutler, W. B., Garcia, C. R., Huggins, G. R., & Lawley, H. J. (1986). Human axillary secretions influence women's menstrual cycles: The role of donor extract of females. *Hormones and Behavior, 20*(4), 474-482. doi: 10.1016/0018-506x(86)90009-7

Prokosch, M. D., Cossa, R. G., Scheib, J. E., & Blozisa, S. A. (2009). Intelligence and mate choice: intelligent men are always appealing. *Evol Human Behav, 30*, 11-20.

Puts, D. A. (2005). Mating context and menstrual phase affect female preferences for male voice pitch. *Evol Hum Behav, 26*, 388-397.

Reber, R., Schwarz, N., & Winkielman, P. (2004). Processing fluency and aesthetic pleasure: is beauty in the perceiver's processing experience? *Pers Soc Psychol Rev, 8*(4), 364-382.

Reid, L. N., & Soley, L. C. (1983). Decorative models and the readership of magazine ads. *Journal of Advertising Research, 23*(2), 27-32.

Richetin, J., Croizet, J.-C., & Huguet, P. (2004). Facial make-up elicits positive attitudes at the implicit level: Evidence from the implicit association test. *Current Research in Social Psychology, 9*(11), No Pagination Specified.

Rieger, G., Linsenmeier, J., Gygax, L., Garcia, S., & Bailey, J. (2010). Dissecting "Gaydar": Accuracy and the Role of Masculinity–Femininity. *Archives of Sexual Behavior, 39*(1), 124-140. doi: 10.1007/s10508-008-9405-2

Rieger, G., Linsenmeier, J. A. W., Gygax, L., & Bailey, J. M. (2008). Sexual orientation and childhood gender nonconformity: Evidence from home videos. *Developmental Psychology, 44*(1), 46-58. doi: 10.1037/0012-1649.44.1.46

Rikowski, A., & Grammer, K. (1999). Human body odour, symmetry and attractiveness. *Proc Biol Sci, 266*(1422), 869-874.

Roberts, S. C., Little, A. C., Gosling, L. M., Jones, B. C., Perrett, D. I., Carter, V., & Petrie, M. (2005). MHC-assortative facial preferences in humans. *Biol Lett, 1*(4), 400-403.

Roizen, M. F., & Puma, J. L. (2002). *The RealAge Diet: Make Yourself Younger with What You Eat*: HarperCollins.

Roll, S., & Verinis, J. S. (1971). Stereotypes of scalp and facial hair as measured by the semantic differential. *Psychological Reports, 28*(3), 975-980.

Rosenbloom, A. L., & Rivkees, S. A. (2010). Off-label use of recombinant igf-I to promote growth: is it appropriate? *J Clin Endocrinol Metab, 95*(2), 505-508.

Roth, T. (1995). An overview of the report of the national commission on sleep disorders research. *European Psychiatry, 10*, Supplement 3(0), 109s-113s. doi: 10.1016/0924-9338(96)80091-5

Rule, N. O., & Ambady, N. (2008). The face of success: inferences from chief executive officers' appearance predict company profits. *Psychol Sci, 19*(2), 109-111. doi: 10.1111/j.1467-9280.2008.02054.x

Rule, N. O., Moran, J. M., Freeman, J. B., Whitfield-Gabrieli, S., Gabrieli, J. D. E., & Ambady, N. (2011). Face value: Amygdala response reflects the validity of first impressions. *NeuroImage, 54*(1), 734-741. doi: 10.1016/j.neuroimage.2010.07.007

Russell, R. (2003). Sex, beauty, and the relative luminance of facial features. *Perception, 32*(9), 1093-1107.

Ryan, A. S., & Goldsmith, L. A. (1996). Nutrition and the skin. *Clin Dermatol, 14*(4), 389-406. doi: 0738-081X(96)00068-5 [pii]

S., B. A., Starzyk, K. B., & Quinsey, V. (2001). The relationship between testosterone and aggression: A meta-analysis. *Aggress Viol Behav, 6*, 579-599.

Sadalla, E. K., Kenrick, K. T., & Vershure, B. (1987). Dominance and heterosexual attraction. *J Pers Soc Psychol, 52*, 730-738.

Sarwer, D. B., Grossbart, T. A., & Didie, E. R. (2003). Beauty and society. *Semin Cutan Med Surg, 22*(2), 79-92. doi: S1085-5629(03)80011-1 [pii] 10.1053/sder.2003.50014

Sell, R. L., Wells, J. A., & Wypij, D. (1995). The prevalence of homosexual behavior and attraction in the United States, the United Kingdom and France: Results of national population-based samples. *Archives of Sexual Behavior, 24*(3), 235-248. doi: 10.1007/bf01541598

Sheldon, J. P., Pfeffer, C. A., Jayaratne, T. E., Feldbaum, M., & Petty, E. M. (2007). Beliefs About the Etiology of Homosexuality and About the Ramifications of Discovering Its Possible Genetic Origin. [Article]. *Journal of Homosexuality, 52*(3/4), 111-150.

Singh, D. (1993). Adaptive significance of female physical attractiveness: role of waist-to-hip ratio. *J Pers Soc Psychol, 65*(2), 293-307.

Slater, A. M., von der Schulenburg, C., Brown, E., Badenoch, M., Butterworth, G., Parsons, S., & Smuels, C. (1998). Newborn infants prefer attractive faces. *Infant Behav Dev, 21*, 345-354.

Small, M. (2011). *What's Love Got to Do with It?* : Knopf Doubleday Publishing Group.

Smith, K. L., Cornelissen, P. L., & Tovée, M. J. (2007). Color 3D bodies and judgements of human female attractiveness. *Evolution and Human Behavior, 28*(1), 48-54. doi: 10.1016/j.evolhumbehav.2006.05.007

Soler, C., Núñez, M., Gutiérrez, R., Núñez, J., Medina, P., Sancho, M., . . . Núñez, A. (2003). Facial attractiveness in men provides clues to semen quality. *Evol Hum Behav, 24*, 199-207.

Springer, I. N., Wannicke, B., Warnke, P. H., Zernial, O., Wiltfang, J., Russo, P. A., . . . Wolfart, S. (2007). Facial attractiveness: visual impact of symmetry increases significantly towards the midline. *Ann Plast Surg, 59*(2), 156-162. doi: 10.1097/01.sap.0000252041.66540.ec

Stephen, I. D., Coetzee, V., Law Smith, M., & Perrett, D. I. (2009). Skin Blood Perfusion and Oxygenation Colour Affect Perceived Human Health. *PLoS One, 4*(4), e5083.

Studer, L. H., Aylwin, A. S., & Reddon, J. R. (2005). Testosterone, sexual offense recidivism, and treatment effect among adult male sex offenders. *Sex Abuse, 17*(2), 171-181.

Surgeons, A. S. o. P. (2005). 2005 ASPS Survey.

Swift A. Remington K. Beuatification a global approach to facial beauty. Clin Plastic Surg 38 (2011) 347. 0

Synnott, A. (1987). Shame and glory: A sociology of hair. *British Journal of Sociology, 38*(3), 381-413. doi: 10.2307/590695

Sypeck, M. F., Gray, J. J., & Ahrens, A. H. (2004). No longer just a pretty face: fashion magazines' depictions of ideal female beauty from 1959 to 1999. *Int J Eat Disord, 36*(3), 342-347.

Thakerar, J. N., & Iwawaki, S. (1979). Cross-cultural comparisons in interpersonal attraction of females toward males. *The Journal of Social Psychology, 108*(1), 121-122.

Thelen, T. H. (1983). Minority type human mate preference. *Biodemography and Social Biology, 30*(2), 162-180.

Thornhill, R., Gangestad, S. W., & Comer, R. (1995). Human female orgasm and mate fluctuating asymmetry. *Animal Behaviour, 50*(6), 1601-1615. doi: 10.1016/0003-3472(95)80014-x

Thornton, M. J. (2002). The biological actions of estrogens on skin. *Exp Dermatol, 11*(6), 487-502.

Thursz, M. R., Thomas, H. C., Greenwood, B. M., & Hill, A. V. (1997). Heterozygote advantage for HLA class-II type in hepatitis B virus infection. *Nat Genet, 17*(1), 11-12.

Todd, P. M., Penke, L., Fasolo, B., & Lenton, A. P. (2007). Different cognitive processes underlie human mate choices and mate preferences. *Proc Natl Acad Sci USA, 104*(38), 15011-15016.

Todorov, A., Mandisodza, A. N., Goren, A., & Hall, C. C. (2005). Inferences of competence from faces predict election outcomes. *Science, 308*(5728), 1623-1626.

Townsend, J. M., & Levy, G. D. (1990). Effects of potential partners' costume and physical attractiveness on sexuality and partner selection. *Journal of Psychology: Interdisciplinary and Applied, 124*(4), 371-389.

van den Berghe, P. L., & Frost, P. (1986). Skin color preference, sexual dimorphism and sexual selection: A case of gene culture co-evolution?*. *Ethnic and Racial Studies, 9*(1), 87-113. doi: 10.1080/01419870.1986.9993516

Voilrath, F., & Milinski, M. (1995). Fragrant genes help Damenwahl. *Trends Ecol Evol, 10*(8), 307-308.

Wade, T. J. (2006). MISSING TITLE. *J Cult Evol Psych, 4*, 37-50.

Wagatsuma, H. (1967). The Social Perception of Skin Color in Japan. *Daedalus, 96*(2), 407-443.

Walker, M., & Vetter, T. (2009). Portraits made to measure: manipulating social judgments about individuals with a statistical face model. *J Vis, 9*(11), 12 11-13. doi: 10.1167/9.11.12

/9/11/12/ [pii]

Wang, C., Swerdloff, R. S., Iranmanesh, A., Dobs, A., Snyder, P. J., Cunningham, G., . . . Berman, N. (2000). Transdermal testosterone gel improves sexual function, mood, muscle strength, and body composition parameters in hypogonadal men. *J Clin Endocrinol Metab, 85*(8), 2839-2853.

Warren, J. M., Henry, C. J. K., & Simonite, V. (2003). Low Glycemic Index Breakfasts and Reduced Food Intake in Preadolescent Children. *Pediatrics, 112*(5), e414. doi: 10.1542/peds.112.5.e414

Wedekind, C., & Füri, S. (1997). Body odour preferences in men and women: do they aim for specific MHC combinations or simply heterozygosity? *Proc Biol Sci, 264*(1387), 1471-1479.

Wedekind, C., Seebeck, T., Bettens, F., & Paepke, A. J. (1995). MHC-dependent mate preferences in humans. *Proc Biol Sci, 260*(1359), 245-249.

Wells, G. L., & Olson, E. A. (2001). The Other-Race Effect in Eyewitness Identification: What Do We Do About It? *Psychology, Public Policy, and Law, 7*(1), 230-246.

White, F. J. (1989). Ecological correlates of pygmy chimpanzee social structure. In V. Standen & R. A. Foley (Eds.), *Comparitive socioecology: The behavioural ecology of humans and other mammals* (pp. 151-164). Boston: Blackwell Scientific Publications.

Willis, J., & Todorov, A. (2006). First impressions: making up your mind after a 100-ms exposure to a face. *Psychol Sci, 17*(7), 592-598. doi: PSCI1750 [pii]

10.1111/j.1467-9280.2006.01750.x

Winston, J. S., O'Doherty, J., Kilner, J. M., Perrett, D. I., & Dolan, R. J. (2007). Brain systems for assessing facial attractiveness. *Neuropsychologia, 45*(1), 195-206.

Wolf, N. (2002). *The beauty myth: how images of beauty are used against women*: Perennial.

Workman, J. E., & Johnson, K. K. P. (1991). The Role of Cosmetics in Impression Formation. *Clothing and Textiles Research Journal, 10*(1), 63-67. doi: 10.1177/0887302x9101000109

Zaadstra, B. M., Seidell, J. C., Van Noord, P. A., te Velde, E. R., Habbema, J. D., Vrieswijk, B., & Karbaat, J. (1993). Fat and female fecundity: prospective study of effect of body fat distribution on conception rates. *BMJ, 306*(6876), 484-487.

Zebrowitz, L. A., & Collins, M. A. (1997). Accurate Social Perception at Zero Acquaintance: The Affordances of a Gibsonian Approach. *Personality and Social Psychology Review, 1*(3), 204-223. doi: 10.1207/s15327957pspr0103_2

Zhou, J.-N., Hofman, M. A., Gooren, L. J. G., & Swaab, D. F. (1995). A sex difference in the human brain and its relation to transsexuality. [10.1038/378068a0]. *Nature, 378*(6552), 68-70.

Zuckerman, M., & Driver, R. E. (1989). What sounds beautiful is good: The vocal attractiveness stereotype. *Journal of Nonverbal Behavior, 13*(2), 67-82. doi: 10.1007/bf00990791

CPSIA information can be obtained at www.ICGtesting.com
Printed in the USA
BVOW081536060513

320015BV00001BA/1/P